Department of Veterans Affairs
Health Services Research & Development Service | Evidence-based Synthesis Program

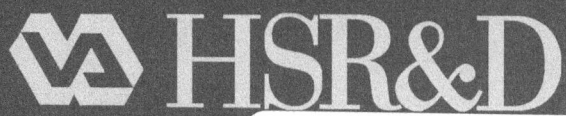

Effects of Care Models to Improve General Medical Outcomes for Individuals With Serious Mental Illness

September 2011

Prepared for:
Department of Veterans Affairs
Veterans Health Administration
Health Services Research & Development Service
Washington, DC 20420

Prepared by:
Evidence-based Synthesis Program (ESP) Center
Durham Veterans Affairs Healthcare System
Durham, NC
John W. Williams Jr., MD, MHSc, Director

Investigators:
Principal Investigator:
  Daniel W. Bradford, MD, MPH

Co-Investigators:
  Monica N. Slubicki, MD
  Jennifer McDuffie, PhD
  Amy Kilbourne, PhD
  John W. Williams Jr., MD, MHSc

Research Associate:
  Avishek Nagi, MS

Medical Editor:
  Liz Wing, MA

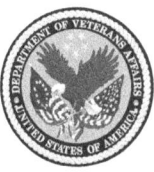

PREFACE

Health Services Research & Development Service's (HSR&D's) Evidence-based Synthesis Program (ESP) was established to provide timely and accurate syntheses of targeted healthcare topics of particular importance to Veterans Affairs (VA) managers and policymakers, as they work to improve the health and healthcare of Veterans. The ESP disseminates these reports throughout VA.

HSR&D provides funding for four ESP Centers and each Center has an active VA affiliation. The ESP Centers generate evidence syntheses on important clinical practice topics, and these reports help:

- develop clinical policies informed by evidence,
- guide the implementation of effective services to improve patient outcomes and to support VA clinical practice guidelines and performance measures, and
- set the direction for future research to address gaps in clinical knowledge.

In 2009, the ESP Coordinating Center was created to expand the capacity of HSR&D Central Office and the four ESP sites by developing and maintaining program processes. In addition, the Center established a Steering Committee comprised of HSR&D field-based investigators, VA Patient Care Services, Office of Quality and Performance, and Veterans Integrated Service Networks (VISN) Clinical Management Officers. The Steering Committee provides program oversight, guides strategic planning, coordinates dissemination activities, and develops collaborations with VA leadership to identify new ESP topics of importance to Veterans and the VA healthcare system.

Comments on this evidence report are welcome and can be sent to Nicole Floyd, ESP Coordinating Center Program Manager, at nicole.floyd@va.gov.

Recommended citation: Bradford DW, Slubicki MN, McDuffie JR, Kilbourne AM, Nagi A, Williams JW Jr. Effects of Care Models to Improve General Medical Outcomes for Individuals With Serious Mental Illness. VA-ESP Project #09-010; 2011

This report is based on research conducted by the Evidence-based Synthesis Program (ESP) Center located at the Durham VA Medical Center, Durham, NC, funded by the Department of Veterans Affairs, Veterans Health Administration, Office of Research and Development, Health Services Research and Development. The findings and conclusions in this document are those of the author(s) who are responsible for its contents; the findings and conclusions do not necessarily represent the views of the Department of Veterans Affairs or the United States government. Therefore, no statement in this article should be construed as an official position of the Department of Veterans Affairs. No investigators have any affiliations or financial involvement (e.g., employment, consultancies, honoraria, stock ownership or options, expert testimony, grants or patents received or pending, or royalties) that conflict with material presented in the report.

TABLE OF CONTENTS

EXECUTIVE SUMMARY
Background 1
Methods 1
Data Synthesis 2
Peer Review 2
Results 2
Abbreviations Table 5

INTRODUCTION
Background 6

METHODS
Topic Development 9
Analytic Framework 9
Search Strategy 10
Study Selection 10
Data Abstraction 12
Quality Assessment 12
Data Synthesis 12
Rating the Body of Evidence 13
Peer Review 13

RESULTS
Literature Flow 14
Study Characteristics 15
KQ 1. What types of care models have been evaluated prospectively that integrate mental health care and primary medical care with the goal of improving general medical outcomes for individuals with serious mental illness (SMI)? 17
KQ 2. Do models of integrated care for individuals with SMI improve the process of care for preventive services (e.g., colorectal cancer screening) and chronic disease management (e.g., annual eye examination in patients with diabetes mellitus [DM])? 20
KQ 3. (3a) Do models of integrated care for individuals with SMI improve general functional status outcomes (e.g., as measured by SF-36) or disease-specific functional status outcomes (e.g., Seattle Angina Questionnaire) related to medical care for chronic medical conditions such as DM, hypertension, or heart failure? (3b) Do models of integrated care for individuals with SMI improve clinical outcomes related to preventive services (e.g., influenza rates) and chronic medical care (e.g., kidney disease, amputations, retinopathy in patients with coexisting DM)? 23
KQ 4. What are the gaps in evidence for determining how best to integrate care to improve general medical outcomes for individuals with SMI? 25

SUMMARY AND DISCUSSION
    Summary of Evidence by Key Question 29
    Limitations 32
    Recommendations for Future Research 33

REFERENCES 35

APPENDIX A. SEARCH STRATEGY 41

APPENDIX B. STUDY SELECTION FORM 42

APPENDIX C. CRITERIA USED IN QUALITY ASSESSMENT 44

APPENDIX D. PEER REVIEW COMMENTS/AUTHOR RESPONSES 46

APPENDIX E. EXCLUDED STUDIES 52

APPENDIX F. GLOSSARY 57

FIGURES
    Figure 1. Analytic framework for general medical outcomes for SMI 10
    Figure 2. Literature flow diagram 14

TABLES
    Table 1.   Summary of inclusion and exclusion criteria 11
    Table 2.   Summary of included studies 16
    Table 3.   SMI intervention characteristics informed by Wagner's Chronic Care Model 18
    Table 4.   Process of care outcomes for preventive care (KQ 2) 22
    Table 5.   Process of care outcomes for chronic disease management (KQ 2) 22
    Table 6.   Outcome measures 24
    Table 7.   Outcome summary for KQ 3 24
    Table 8.   Summary of gaps in evidence 25
    Table 9.   Ongoing studies evaluating integrated approaches 28
    Table 10. Strength of evidence by key question 29
    Table 11. Quality assessment for the four RCTs 45

EXECUTIVE SUMMARY

BACKGROUND

Individuals with serious mental illness (SMI) have shortened life expectancies relative to the general population to an extent that is not explained by unnatural causes such as suicide or accidents. Numerous studies show higher rates of acute and chronic illnesses, lower quality general medical care and worse outcomes in individuals with SMI. The issues that influence general medical outcomes for individuals with SMI are complex and overlapping and likely vary by disease state. Relevant factors can be categorized to include population characteristics, contextual and system factors, provider factors, and community resources. Interventions aimed at improving general medical outcomes in this population could be directed at any one, or several, of these factors. The organization of service delivery for individuals with SMI may be the most modifiable of the many factors that impact general medical outcomes in this population. In this review, we sought to evaluate models of care designed to improve general medical outcomes among individuals with SMI. We conducted a systematic review of the peer-reviewed literature to answer the following key questions (KQs):

KQ 1. What types of care models have been evaluated prospectively that integrate mental health care and primary medical care with the goal of improving general medical outcomes for individuals with serious mental illness (SMI)?

KQ 2. Do models of integrated care for individuals with SMI improve the process of care for preventive services (e.g., colorectal cancer screening) and chronic disease management (e.g., annual eye examination in patients with diabetes mellitus [DM])?

KQ 3. (3a) Do models of integrated care for individuals with SMI improve general functional status outcomes (e.g., as measured by SF-36) or disease-specific functional status outcomes (e.g., Seattle Angina Questionnaire) related to medical care for chronic medical conditions such as DM, hypertension, or heart failure? (3b) Do models of integrated care for individuals with SMI improve clinical outcomes related to preventive services (e.g., influenza rates) and chronic medical care (e.g., kidney disease, amputations, retinopathy in patients with coexisting DM)?

KQ 4. What are the gaps in evidence for determining how best to integrate care to improve general medical outcomes for individuals with SMI?

This review was commissioned by the Department of Veterans Affairs' Evidence-based Synthesis Program. The topic was selected after a formal topic nomination and prioritization process that included representatives from the Office of Mental Health Services, Health Services Research and Development, the Mental Health Quality Enhancement Research Initiative (QUERI), and the Office of Mental Health and Primary Care Integration.

METHODS

We searched for English-language publications in MEDLINE® (via PubMed®), Embase®, PsycINFO®, and the Cochrane Library from database inception through March 10, 2011. Search terms included terms for schizophrenia and bipolar disorder; a broad set of terms for care models; and a set of terms for randomized controlled trials (RCTs) or quasi-experimental studies adapted from the Cochrane Effective Practice and Organization of Care Search. We supplemented electronic searching by examining the bibliographies of the included studies and other review articles. Finally, we searched ClinicalTrials.gov using the terms "serious mental illness" or "SMI" to assess for evidence of publication bias (completed but unpublished studies) and ongoing studies that may fill gaps in evidence.

Titles, abstracts, and articles were reviewed in duplicate by investigators trained in the critical analysis of literature. To be included in our evidence report, a study had to (1) be a randomized controlled trial (RCT) or quasi-experimental study design, (2) evaluate a care model designed to integrate mental and general medical care, (3) include a sample of adult patients with SMI (i.e., schizophrenia, bipolar disorder, schizoaffective disorder) or who met the definition of SMI based on low functional status (e.g., by Global Assessment of Functioning score), and (4) report a relevant outcome. Study characteristics, patient characteristics, and outcomes were extracted by trained research staff. We assessed the risk of bias pertaining to KQs 2 and 3 using the key quality criteria described in the Agency for Healthcare Research and Quality (AHRQ) *Methods Guide for Effectiveness and Comparative Effectiveness Reviews*: adequacy of randomization and allocation concealment, comparability of groups at baseline, blinding, completeness of followup and differential loss to followup, whether incomplete data were addressed appropriately, validity of outcome measures and completeness of outcomes reporting, and conflict of interest.

DATA SYNTHESIS

We constructed summary tables showing the study characteristics and results for all included studies, organized by KQ. We critically analyzed studies to compare their characteristics, methods, and findings. We compiled a summary of findings for each KQ and drew conclusions based on qualitative synthesis of the findings. There were not sufficient studies to perform quantitative synthesis (meta-analysis). We graded the strength of evidence for KQ 2 and KQ3 using principles from the Grades of Recommendation, Assessment, Development, and Evaluation (GRADE) Working Group. This approach assesses the strength of evidence for each critical outcome by considering risk of bias, consistency, directness, precision, and publication bias. After considering each domain, a summary rating of "high," "moderate," "low," or "insufficient" strength of evidence was assigned.

PEER REVIEW

This draft version of the report will be reviewed by technical experts as well as clinical leadership, and their comments will be considered in the final report.

RESULTS

We reviewed 1598 titles and abstracts from the electronic search and an additional 24 from reference mining for a total of 1622 references. After applying inclusion/exclusion criteria at the abstract level, 1565 references were excluded. We retrieved 57 full-text articles for further review, after which another 50 articles were excluded. We identified a total of seven articles for inclusion in the current review, representing four RCTs. No non-RCT studies met eligibility criteria.

Of the four RCTs, three were set in the VA facilities and one was set in a community mental health center. Because two studies focused entirely on individuals with bipolar disorder, the proportion of subjects with other SMIs was relatively low, with just 19 percent of the overall samples identified as having schizophrenia or schizoaffective disorder.

KQ 1. What types of care models have been evaluated prospectively that integrate mental health care and primary medical care with the goal of improving general medical outcomes for individuals with serious mental illness (SMI)?

Four RCTs evaluated approaches to integrated care; most studies were theoretically based on Wagner's Chronic Care Model. All integrated care models were set in mental health specialty settings, added new personnel, and used care management or care coordination as a key strategy. Only one study used co-located mental health and general medical services. Self-management support was a component in three of the four studies, but only one study used decision support for general medical care. On the spectrum of limited integration (e.g., communication between providers) to fully integrated (e.g., shared development and implementation of the treatment plan), the interventions tested range from limited to moderately integrated.

The four studies represented in our review were similar in many ways, showing a relatively limited variety of approaches to improving general medical care for individuals with SMI. Notably, professionals such as psychologists, with expertise in facilitating behavior change, and nutritionists were not incorporated into the models tested. As described above, three of the four studies had substantial basis in the Chronic Care Model, but elements of the patient-centered medical home (PCMH), such as having a primary treating provider, team-based care, and enhanced access, were not robustly employed.

KQ 2. Do models of integrated care for individuals with SMI improve the process of care for preventive services (e.g., colorectal cancer screening) and chronic disease management (e.g., annual eye examination in patients with diabetes mellitus [DM])?

Two good-quality RCTs involving 527 patients reported outcomes relevant to this question. Compared to usual care, interventions showed generally positive effects on immunization rates, cancer screening, and selected screening for cardiovascular disease in nonintegrated care systems. We rated the strength of evidence for these outcomes as moderate. However, some measures represented a "low bar," such as measuring weight rather than evaluating the quality of care for weight control, and important cancer-screening practices (e.g., mammography, pap smears) and chronic disease care unrelated to cardiovascular disease were not studied.

KQ 3. (3a) Do models of integrated care for individuals with SMI improve general functional status outcomes (e.g., as measured by SF-36) or disease-specific functional status outcomes (e.g., Seattle Angina Questionnaire) related to medical care for chronic medical conditions such as DM, hypertension, or heart failure? (3b) Do models of integrated care for individuals with SMI improve clinical outcomes related to preventive services (e.g., influenza rates) and chronic medical care (e.g., kidney disease, amputations, retinopathy in patients with coexisting DM)?

Four good-quality RCTs, involving 891 subjects, reported effects on functional status outcomes, but no studies reported effects on clinical outcomes. Compared to usual care, integrated care in two RCTs showed small, statistically significant improvements in physical functioning at followup periods ranging from 12 to 52 weeks. Two other RCTs did not find statistically significant differences using similar health outcome survey measures when comparing integrated care to usual care. Thus, effects on physical function appear small and inconsistent. However, interventions varied in their focus on care processes that could be expected to improve physical function. Followup periods ranged from 26 to 156 weeks, and interventions that focused primarily on preventive care could be expected to require long followup periods in order to show positive effects on physical functioning. Interventions that are more tailored to specific disease states or that utilize greater levels of integration and organizational support may be required to produce more robust effects on functional status.

Three of the four studies were conducted in the VA system, with two of three VA studies demonstrating improvements in physical functioning. Given the range of medical services generally offered on site at VA healthcare locations, integration and collocation approaches may be easier to implement in VHA than many other health care systems.

KQ 4. What are the gaps in evidence for determining how best to integrate care to improve general medical outcomes for individuals with SMI?

Among the four studies reviewed, there was relatively little diversity in the types of models tested, with most models based on Wagner's Chronic Care Model. Elements of PCMH, other than those that overlap with the chronic care model, were not generally evaluated. Given the high prevalence of cardiovascular disease in individuals with SMI, the focus on process of care for cardiovascular disease is important. However, effects of integrated care on a broader range of preventive and chronic disease services and, importantly, clinical outcomes is needed. Finally, relatively few individuals with schizophrenia and related psychotic disorders were included in these studies, and it is uncertain if the positive effects would be replicated in these patients.

Our search of ClinicalTrials.gov found three ongoing RCTs and one ongoing non-RCT evaluating care models for individuals with SMI.

The following table summarizes the key gaps in evidence.

Key gaps in evidence

The key intervention components are uncertain.
There is greater uncertainty about intervention effects for individuals with SMIs other than bipolar disorder.
Effects on clinical outcomes have not been studied.
Sustainability of intervention effects is uncertain.
Effects of interventions (effectiveness) are uncertain when part of routine care rather than part of an RCT.
Effects of current VA delivery models are uncertain, including primary care services co-located in the mental health setting and assertive community treatment.
There is uncertainty about effects of current VA programs to improve mental health outcomes of veterans with SMI (e.g., assertive community treatment) that theoretically may have beneficial effects on general medical outcomes.

ABBREVIATIONS TABLE

AHRQ	Agency for Healthcare Research and Quality
DM	diabetes mellitus
KQ	key question
MeSH	medical subject headings
PCMH	patient-centered medical home
RCT	randomized controlled trial
SMI	serious mental illness
VA	Veterans Affairs
VHA	Veterans Health Administration

EVIDENCE REPORT

INTRODUCTION

Individuals with serious mental illness (SMI) have shortened life expectancies relative to the general population[1,2] to an extent that is not explained by unnatural causes such as suicide or accidents. Epidemiological studies have estimated the life expectancy of individuals with schizophrenia to be 10 to 25 years less than the general population.[3-6] Increased morbidity of both chronic and acute illnesses in individuals with SMI also reduces quality of life and increases the overall burden of disability beyond that of the SMI itself. SMIs have an overwhelming economic impact, as measured by direct and indirect costs, including health care costs, disability payments, lost productivity, and law enforcement costs. For example, one study estimated annual costs due to schizophrenia to be $62.7 billion annually in the U.S.,[7] and patients with bipolar disorder are estimated to have the highest total health care costs of any mental illness[8,9] with up to 70 percent of these costs in non–mental health (e.g., primary care) settings.[10,11] Given these issues, methods to improve general medical services for individuals with SMI is a pressing priority.

BACKGROUND

The issues that influence general medical outcomes for individuals with SMI are complex and overlapping and likely vary by disease state. Relevant factors can be categorized to include population characteristics, contextual and system factors, provider factors, and community resources. Interventions aimed at improving general medical outcomes in this population could be directed at any one, or several, of these factors.

The populations of individuals with SMI have consistently shown higher rates of illnesses, such as infectious disease,[12] diabetes,[13-15] respiratory illness,[16] and cardiovascular disease,[17,18] than the general population. Modifiable risk factors for poor health, such as smoking,[19] obesity,[20,21] alcohol and substance abuse,[22] and lack of exercise,[23] are highly prevalent in individuals with SMI—as are obstacles to optimal health care such as poverty,[24] homelessness,[25] and social isolation.[26]

Multiple studies show diminished guideline concordance of general medical care provided to individuals with SMI, as evidenced by reduced receipt of preventive medical services[27,28] and lower quality of chronic disease management for illnesses such as diabetes[29,30] and cardiovascular disease[31] as well as acute illnesses such as myocardial infarction.[32] In addition, psychiatric medications can be risk factors for poor health given the association with some pharmacological treatments and medical outcomes such as increased risk of sudden death,[33] hyperglycemia,[34] hyperlipidemia,[35] and weight gain.[36]

Effectiveness of Health Care Providers

The effectiveness of health care providers in optimizing general medical outcomes in individuals with SMI depends on multiple factors, including the type and level of training for working with this complex population, attitudes and beliefs about individuals with SMI, and knowledge of specific issues affecting individuals with SMI. The range of professionals involved with providing psychiatric care to patients with SMI includes disciplines with little or no training in medical issues. Among physician mental health providers (i.e., psychiatrists), general medical training is typically limited to less than 6 months of direct service in internal medicine settings. Further, general medical providers usually have limited experience working with patients with SMI. Although combined training programs, such as those in psychiatry and internal medicine, produce physicians who are well trained to address both medical and psychiatric problems, there are relatively few of these programs—only 17 in the U.S.[37]—so graduates of such programs represent a small minority of those who provide general medical services along with SMI care.

Settings of Care

The characteristics of various sites of care where individuals with SMI receive general medical services affect the general medical outcomes of this population. Individuals with SMI may receive psychiatric and general medical care at sites separated by geography, organization, financing, and/or culture.[38] While integration of mental health and primary care services has been implemented in some settings for depressive and anxiety disorders, general medical and psychiatric services typically are received at different sites for individuals with SMI. Payment structures may not incentivize collaboration of care among medical and psychiatric care providers, making the increased time challenging for this important element of care. Even in integrated systems with single payers, medical and psychiatric care systems may be held accountable for outcomes that sometimes lead to conflicting medical decisions (e.g., psychotropic medication choice may lead to improved psychiatric symptom control while worsening metabolic indices).

Supportive Services

A further impact to general medical outcomes in persons with SMI may be the availability of various types of supportive services that facilitate overall well-being and access to care. While it has not been systematically studied to this point, the availability of housing, intensive case management services, and employment support would be expected to positively influence adherence to recommendations and the ability of persons with SMI to access general medical care.

Integration of Care

In this evidence synthesis, we sought to elucidate the best ways to integrate medical and mental health care to improve general medical outcomes in individuals with SMI. We were interested in understanding methods of integration of care for those whose psychiatric disability causes the greatest barriers to general medical care and for whom the site of greatest interaction with health care is the psychiatric setting. The term "serious mental illness" has been defined multiple ways and includes groupings of diagnoses and ratings of functional impairment, such as the Global Assessment of Functioning. Because the rating of illness severity—particularly those elements (e.g., cognitive functioning, communication abilities) that are most likely to have an impact on the quality of general medical healthcare received—is rarely reported in studies of general medical care in persons with SMI, we used reported psychiatric diagnoses as the best available proxy.

For this review, we chose to focus on the mental disorders of schizophrenia, schizoaffective disorder, and bipolar disorder as representative of the more serious mental illnesses. Lending support to this decision are the results of an analysis of a nationally representative survey[39] showing that individuals with psychotic disorders and bipolar disorder, but not major depression, were less likely than the general population to have a primary care provider even after controlling for demographics, income, and insurance status. Another factor in this choice was the large body of literature[40,41] and subsequent reviews[42,43] that have described efforts to integrate primary and mental health care for individuals with unipolar depression and anxiety disorders.

Throughout health care systems, including the Veterans Health Administration (VHA), there is increasing emphasis on the patient-centered medical home (PCMH);[44,45] however, the ways this model will be implemented in the care of individuals with SMI remain unclear. The organization of service delivery for individuals with SMI may be the most modifiable of the many factors that impact general medical outcomes in this population. In addition, components may be added to the delivery of care to enhance medical outcomes, such as patient self-management interventions, decision support, and shared medical records. In this review, we sought to evaluate models of care designed to improve general medical outcomes among individuals with SMI.

METHODS

TOPIC DEVELOPMENT

This review was commissioned by the Department of Veterans Affairs' Evidence-based Synthesis Program. The topic was selected after a formal topic nomination and prioritization process that included representatives from the Office of Mental Health Services, Health Services Research and Development, the Mental Health Quality Enhancement Research Initiative (QUERI), and the Office of Mental Health and Primary Care Integration.

The final key questions (KQs) were:

KQ 1. What types of care models have been evaluated prospectively that integrate mental health care and primary medical care with the goal of improving general medical outcomes for individuals with serious mental illness (SMI)?

KQ 2. Do models of integrated care for individuals with SMI improve the process of care for preventive services (e.g., colorectal cancer screening) and chronic disease management (e.g., annual eye examination in patients with diabetes mellitus [DM])?

KQ 3. (3a) Do models of integrated care for individuals with SMI improve general functional status outcomes (e.g., as measured by SF-36) or disease-specific functional status outcomes (e.g., Seattle Angina Questionnaire) related to medical care for chronic medical conditions such as DM, hypertension, or heart failure? (3b) Do models of integrated care for individuals with SMI improve clinical outcomes related to preventive services (e.g., influenza rates) and chronic medical care (e.g., kidney disease, amputations, retinopathy in patients with coexisting DM)?

KQ 4. What are the gaps in evidence for determining how best to integrate care to improve general medical outcomes for individuals with SMI?

ANALYTIC FRAMEWORK

We developed and followed a standard protocol for all steps of this review. Our approach was guided by an analytic framework adapted from a previously developed behavioral model for vulnerable populations.[46] Figure 1 shows the analytic framework.

Figure 1. Analytic framework for general medical outcomes for SMI

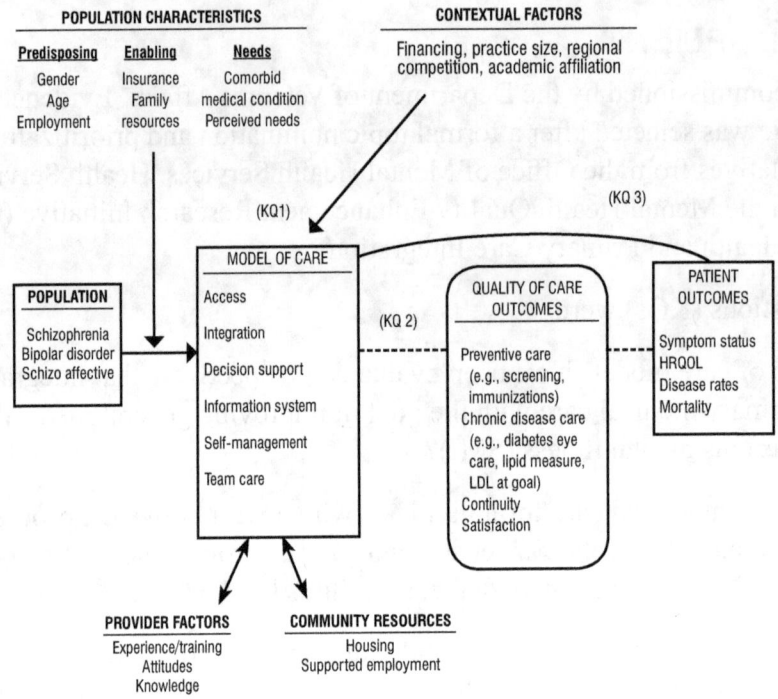

SEARCH STRATEGY

We searched for English-language publications in MEDLINE® (via PubMed®), Embase®, PsycINFO®, and the Cochrane Library from database inception through March 10, 2011. Search terms included terms for schizophrenia and bipolar disorder; a broad set of terms for care models; and a set of terms for randomized controlled trials (RCTs) or quasi-experimental studies adapted from the Cochrane Effective Practice and Organization of Care Search.[47-50] The search strategies were developed in consultation with a master librarian. The search terms and MeSH headings for the search strategies appear in Appendix A. We supplemented electronic searching by examining the bibliographies of the included studies and other review articles. Finally, we searched ClinicalTrials.gov using the terms "serious mental illness" or "SMI" to assess for evidence of publication bias (completed but unpublished studies) and ongoing studies that may fill gaps in evidence.

STUDY SELECTION

Using prespecified inclusion/exclusion criteria (Appendix B), two reviewers assessed the lists of titles and abstracts from the databases for further review. Full-text articles of potentially relevant abstracts were retrieved for further review. To be included in our evidence report, a study had to (1) be a randomized controlled trial (RCT) or quasi-experimental study design, (2) evaluate a care model designed to integrate mental and general medical care, (3) include a sample of adult patients with SMI (i.e., schizophrenia, bipolar disorder, schizoaffective disorder) or who met the definition of SMI based on low functional status (e.g., by Global Assessment of Functioning score) and (4) report a relevant outcome. If both preliminary and final reports were published, the final data analysis was utilized. The eligibility criteria are described in detail in Table 1.

Table 1. Summary of inclusion and exclusion criteria

Study characteristic	Inclusion criteria	Exclusion criteria
Study design	RCT or quasi-experimental study defined as nonrandomized cluster controlled trial, controlled before-and-after study, or interrupted time series	Non-English language publication Cross-sectional and other observational designs not listed as included
Population	Adults ≥ 18 years of age with schizophrenia, schizoaffective disorder, or bipolar disorder A sample described as persons having SMI (based on low functional status and chronicity) and at least 25% are diagnosed with schizophrenia, schizoaffective disorder, or bipolar disorder	Primary substance abuse
Interventions	Interventions with a stated goal to improve general medical care or outcomes through an integrated model and either one of the following: (1) a system redesign that adds care provider(s) to directly address or coordinate mental and general medical care (2) interventions that do not add providers but include at least 3 of the following elements: • decision support • information systems • self-management support • team care • enhanced communications between mental health providers and general medical providers	Interventions designed to be implemented primarily in the community (nonmedical settings) Interventions designed to affect only one specific outcome or aspect of general medical health (e.g., weight loss or smoking cessation, etc.)
Comparators	Usual care or other quality improvement strategy	None
Outcomes	Process of care measures for preventive services (e.g., influenza vaccination rate), or chronic disease management (e.g., lipid screening or glucose control in a patient with diabetes mellitus) Clinical outcomes (e.g., rate of influenza infection) Physical functioning (SF-36 Physical Component) or disease-specific symptoms (e.g., Seattle Angina Questionnaire) measured by a validated instrument	Only measures of mental health care processes, symptom status, or functional status
Setting	Outpatient mental health	Hospital-based (inpatient) settings Community-based settings (e.g., senior centers, homeless shelters)

DATA ABSTRACTION

A trained researcher abstracted data from published articles and reports into a data abstraction form; a second reviewer overread the abstracted data. We resolved disagreements by consensus among the first and second reviewer or by obtaining a third reviewer's opinion when consensus could not be reached. We abstracted the following data for each included study:

- study design
- setting
- population characteristics
- subject eligibility and exclusion criteria
- number of subjects and providers
- intervention(s)
- comparison(s)
- length of followup
- outcome(s)

Intervention characteristics were categorized using the chronic care model and selected elements of the patient centered medical home. The chronic care model classifies health care elements into six domains: health system, delivery system design, decision support, clinical information systems, self-management support, and the community.[51] With the exception of health system factors (e.g., quality-based incentives), we used these domains along with the following PCMH elements: a primary treating clinician, team-based care, and methods to enhance access to care.

We grouped immunizations and cancer screening into the general category of preventive services outcomes. For chronic disease care processes, we prioritized those with an established link to clinical outcomes (e.g., blood pressure control in patients with diabetes mellitus). Some care processes (e.g., cholesterol measurement) could be classified as preventive screening or chronic disease management. When these outcomes were reported separately, we grouped them according to our analytic framework, but in some cases we could not follow this approach because preventive and chronic disease outcomes were reported only in aggregate form.

QUALITY ASSESSMENT

We assessed the risk of bias pertaining to KQs 2 and 3 using the key quality criteria described in the Agency for Healthcare Research and Quality (AHRQ) *Methods Guide for Effectiveness and Comparative Effectiveness Reviews*,[52] adapted for this specific topic (Appendix C). For RCTs, we abstracted data on adequacy of randomization and allocation concealment, comparability of groups at baseline, blinding, completeness of followup and differential loss to followup, whether incomplete data were addressed appropriately, validity of outcome measures and completeness of outcomes reporting, and conflict of interest. Using these data elements, we assigned a summary quality score of Good, Fair, or Poor to individual RCTs. We assessed studies for applicability to U.S. Veterans.

DATA SYNTHESIS

We constructed summary tables showing the study characteristics and results for all included studies, organized by KQ, intervention, or clinical condition, as appropriate. We critically analyzed studies to compare their characteristics, methods, and findings. We compiled a summary of findings for each KQ or clinical topic and drew conclusions based on qualitative synthesis of the findings. There were not sufficient studies to perform quantitative synthesis (meta-analysis).

RATING THE BODY OF EVIDENCE

We assessed the overall quality of evidence for outcomes using a method developed by the Grades of Recommendation, Assessment, Development, and Evaluation (GRADE) Working Group,[53] which classified the grade of evidence across outcomes according to the following criteria:

- High—Further research is very unlikely to change our confidence on the estimate of effect.
- Moderate—Further research is likely to have an important impact on our confidence in the estimate of effect and may change the estimate.
- Low—Further research is very likely to have an important impact on our confidence in the estimate of effect and is likely to change the estimate.
- Insufficient—Evidence on an outcome is absent or too weak, sparse, or inconsistent to estimate an effect.

PEER REVIEW

A draft version of this report was reviewed by technical experts as well as clinical leadership, and their comments are provided in Appendix D.

RESULTS

LITERATURE FLOW

We reviewed 1598 titles and abstracts from the electronic search and an additional 24 from reference mining for a total of 1622 references. After applying inclusion/exclusion criteria at the abstract level, 1565 references were excluded. We retrieved 57 full-text articles for further review, after which another 50 articles were excluded. We identified a total of seven articles for inclusion in the current review, representing four RCTs. Four articles contained the main outcomes of the RCTs, and three articles, referred to as "companion articles," contained additional data pertinent to the four RCTs. We grouped the studies by KQ. Figure 2 details the exclusion criteria at the full-text level and the number of articles related to each of the KQs.

Additionally, our search of www.clinicaltrials.gov identified 208 potentially relevant trials. Of these, four were RCTs and one was a non-RCT of integrated care treatments for individuals with SMI. One of these trials was completed, published, and identified in our MEDLINE search.[54] The other four studies have yet to be completed. Since we did not identify any registered and completed but unpublished trials, there was no evidence in this database of publication bias. The identified trial studies, along with one additional observational study identified through contacts with experts, are summarized in KQ 4.

Figure 2 illustrates each step of our literature search process. Appendix E provides a complete listing of articles excluded at the full-text stage, with reasons for exclusion.

Figure 2. Literature flow diagram

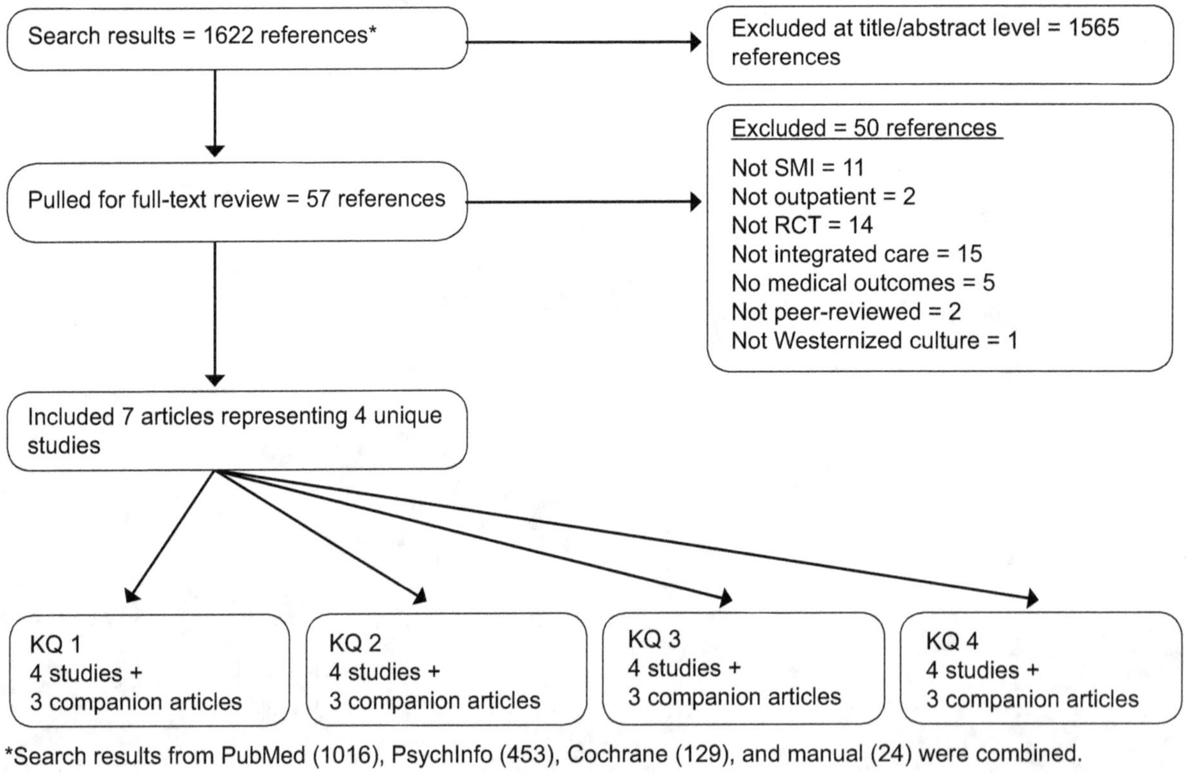

```
Search results = 1622 references*  ───▶  Excluded at title/abstract level = 1565 references
           │
           ▼
                                          Excluded = 50 references
                                          Not SMI = 11
Pulled for full-text review = 57  ───▶    Not outpatient = 2
references                                Not RCT = 14
           │                              Not integrated care = 15
           ▼                              No medical outcomes = 5
                                          Not peer-reviewed = 2
Included 7 articles representing          Not Westernized culture = 1
4 unique studies
      │        │        │        │
      ▼        ▼        ▼        ▼
   KQ 1     KQ 2     KQ 3     KQ 4
  4 studies + 4 studies + 4 studies + 4 studies +
  3 companion 3 companion 3 companion 3 companion
  articles    articles    articles    articles
```

*Search results from PubMed (1016), PsychInfo (453), Cochrane (129), and manual (24) were combined.

Abbreviations: KQ = key question; RCT = randomized controlled trial; SMI = serious mental illness

STUDY CHARACTERISTICS

Basic characteristics of the included studies are summarized in Table 2. Four good-quality RCTs (891subjects) met eligibility criteria; no quasi-experimental studies met eligibility criteria. The psychiatric diagnoses of interest (schizophrenia, schizoaffective disorder, and bipolar disorder) varied in proportion in each study, with two samples[55-59] entirely consisting of patients with bipolar disorder and another sample[60] with 21 to 34 percent carrying the diagnoses of interest. Another study[54] included 49 percent with the diagnoses of interest. Druss and colleagues (2001)[54] reported that 72 to 80 percent of the sample had "severe psychiatric illness" as defined by criteria of the National Advisory Mental Health Council.[61]

Three studies[54,57,59,60] tested interventions specifically aimed at improving general medical outcomes, while one study[55] focused primarily on psychiatric pathology but included an emphasis on primary care enrollment and collaboration. Care management or care coordination was a common element in the studies; only one study employed co-location of medical and psychiatric services.

Three studies[55,57,59,60] were conducted in VA outpatient mental health settings, and one study was conducted in an urban community mental health center.[54] Samples in VA settings had relatively few female participants (ranging from 0.8 to 29%) while almost one-half the sample was female in the urban community mental health center study. Participants were, on average, mid-life adults; mean ages ranged from 47 to 55 years of age. Followup varied from 24 to 156 weeks. A summary of the detailed quality assessment of the studies is found in Appendix C.

Effects of Care Models to Improve General Medical Outcomes for Individuals With Serious Mental Illness

Table 2. Summary of included studies

Study	Design	Subjects		Setting	Intervention summary	Followup	General medical outcomes	Quality
		Disorder	*Demographics*					
Druss et al., 2001[60]	RCT with usual care control N = 120	Schizophrenia: 21% PTSD: 29% Major affective disorder: 13% Substance use: 28% "Severe psychiatric illness" by NAMHC criteria: 76%	Gender: 0.8% female Mean age (yr): 45.2 +/- 8.2 Race: 70% white	VA outpatient mental health	Co-located general medical clinic with care provided by a nurse practitioner with supervision from a family practitioner. Care coordination provided by a nurse.	52 wk	U.S. Preventive Services Task Force indicators; general medical service use	Good
Bauer et al., 2006[55,56] Kilbourne et al., 2009[58] (VA Cooperative Study)	RCT with usual care control N = 306	Bipolar disorder type I: 87% Bipolar disorder type II: 13%	Gender: 28% female Mean age (yr): 46.6 +/- 10.1 Race: 71% "minority"	VA outpatient mental health	Specialty team of psychiatrist and nurse care manager, including self-management support, decision support, emphasis on primary care enrollment and collaboration	156 wk	SF-36 Physical Health	Good
Kilbourne et al., 2008[57,59]	RCT with usual care control N = 58	Bipolar disorder type I: 76% Bipolar disorder type II: 7% Bipolar disorder NOS: 17%	Gender: 9% female Mean age (yr): 55.3+/- 8.4 Race: 10% African American	VA outpatient mental health	Bipolar disorder medical care model consisting of 4 sessions self-management support, nurse care management, guideline implementation related to cardiovascular risk factors	24 wk	SF-12 quality of life-physical health; WHO-DAS	Good
Druss et al., 2010[54]	RCT with usual care control N = 407	Schizophrenia/schizoaffective disorder: 36.4% Bipolar disorder: 13.1% PTSD: 5.1% Depression: 45.2% Other: 0.3% Co-occurring substance use disorder: 26%	Gender: 48.4% female Mean age (yr): 46.7 +/- 8.1 Race: 77.4% African American Hispanic or Latino: 1.5% White: 21.1%	Urban community mental health center	Nurse care management with self-management, liaison, and case management components	52 wk	RAND Community Quality Index; SF-36; Framingham Cardiac Index	Good

Abbreviations: NAMHC = National Advisory Mental Health Council; PTSD = posttraumatic stress disorder; RCT = randomized controlled trial; SF-36 = Short Form-36; VA = Veterans Affairs; WHO-DAS = World Health Organization–Disability Assessment Schedule; wk = week/weeks

KEY QUESTION 1. What types of care models have been evaluated prospectively that integrate mental health care and primary medical care with the goal of improving general medical outcomes for individuals with serious mental illness (SMI)?

Studies of Efficacy

Our review identified four RCTs that met our inclusion criteria. Classification of the models of care used in these studies was informed by Wagner's Chronic Care model.[51,62-64] The models of care used in two studies[55-59] were explicitly based on Wagner's model. A third study [54] also utilized these principles, while the fourth study[60] did not state a clear theoretical model on which it was based.

As required in our inclusion criteria, all the interventions were based primarily in a mental health setting, but integration of general medical services varied from services contiguous with the mental health clinic[60] to care management provided from remote locations.[55-59] Three studies[54-59] relied on research funds to pay the key staff used for the study intervention, while one study[60] was conducted in a setting where the psychiatry service paid the salaries of the staff involved in the intervention through clinical funds. The spectrum of clinical disciplines employed in the interventions of the four RCTs was relatively narrow and limited to those trained traditionally with a primary biomedical orientation (e.g., physicians, nurses, nurse practitioners). All the study interventions employed team-based care—at least to the extent of collaboration by multiple providers to help patients with their mental health and general medical problems. None of the studies used fully integrated teams of mental health and general medical providers working closely together with regular team meetings.

In Table 3 and the paragraphs that follow, each intervention is summarized relative to the components of Wagner's Chronic Care Model.

Table 3. SMI intervention characteristics informed by Wagner's Chronic Care Model

Study	Primary provider	Model elements						
		Team-based	Enhanced access	Self-management support	Decision support	Delivery system	Information systems	Community linkages
Druss et al., 2001[60]	Primary care: yes Psychiatric care: per usual care procedures	Supervising family practitioner and nurse practitioner; liaison with mental health providers	Primary care appointments scheduled to immediately follow mental health appointments when possible	None reported	None reported	Co-location of mental health and primary care services	VA computerized record (both study arms)	None reported
Bauer et al., 2006[55,56] Kilbourne et al., 2009[58] (VA Cooperative Study)	Primary care: per usual care procedures Psychiatric care: nurse care manager for bipolar disorder specific care; otherwise per usual care procedures	Primary care: emphasis on primary care enrollment and collaboration; otherwise per usual care procedures Psychiatric care: "specialty team" comprised of a psychiatrist and nurse care coordinator	Nurse care manager provided same day telephone and next business day clinic appointments	Psychoeducational program (Life Goals Program) primarily addressing bipolar disorder symptoms	Simplified VA Bipolar Clinical Practice Guidelines for providers	Care management; Bipolar Disorders Program	VA computerized record (both study arms)	None reported
Kilbourne et al., 2008[57,59]	Primary care: per usual care procedures Psychiatric care: nurse care manager as first response for bipolar disorder specific care; otherwise per usual care procedures	Nurse care manager provided liaison between existing providers	None reported	Four-session group lead by nurse care manager	Continuing medical education and guidelines; pocket cards for medical and mental health providers related to cardiovascular risk factor management	Care management; Bipolar Disorder Medical Care Model	VA computerized record (both study arms)	None reported
Druss et al., 2010[54]	Primary care and mental health care: per usual care procedures	Nurse care manager provided liaison between mental health and medical providers	None reported	Care manager provided motivational interviewing, development of action plans, and coaching	None reported	Care management	None reported	Public transportation and child care

Abbreviations: VA = Veterans Affairs

Druss and colleagues (2001)[60] conducted a good-quality RCT evaluating a co-located, integrated medical clinic contiguous with the existing mental health outpatient clinic versus usual care in a VA medical center. Continuity of primary medical care was provided by a team that included a nurse practitioner who was supervised by a family practitioner, a nurse case manager, and an administrative assistant. The family practitioner acted as a liaison between the physicians in the medical and psychiatry services. Enhanced access was provided by reminder calls, followup after missed appointments, and efforts to schedule primary care visits immediately following mental health visits. Providers in both the intervention and usual care arms of the study had access to the VA's electronic medical record system including records from all care in the VA system. The study intervention did not include additional decision support or community linkages. This study intervention was not reported as being designed according to an explicitly stated theoretical model.

Investigators in the VA Cooperative Study[55,56,58] conducted a multisite, good-quality RCT to evaluate the effectiveness of the Bipolar Collaborative Chronic Care Model versus usual care in 11 VA medical centers. The delivery system was a "specialty team" located in the outpatient mental health setting and consisted of a psychiatrist who worked in collaboration with the nurse care coordinator. The nurse care coordinator provided enhanced access to mental health care with same-day telephone visits and next-business-day clinic visits. While focused primarily on management of bipolar disorder symptoms, the study intervention also emphasized enrollment in primary care and collaboration with medical providers [55] utilizing the nurse care manager. Self-management support, focused on bipolar disorder, was provided through a psychoeducational group (Life Goals Program) led by the nurse care coordinator over the first year of the intervention. Decision support, again primarily related to bipolar disorder, was implemented by providing the psychiatrists a one-page summary and a six-page manual of the VA Bipolar Clinical Practice Guidelines. Providers in both the intervention and usual care arms of the study had access to the VA's electronic medical record system. The study intervention did not include community linkages. This study intervention was based on Wagner's Chronic Care Model and also drew on elements from the PCMH with a stated patient-centered focus on care for bipolar disorder.

Kilbourne and colleagues (2008)[57,59] conducted a good-quality RCT that evaluated an intervention using existing services for medical and psychiatric care in a VA medical center mental health outpatient setting augmented by the bipolar disorder medical care model, emphasizing self-management, care management, and guidelines implementation compared to usual care. The intervention began with providing four 3-hour sessions aimed at enhancing self-management of bipolar disorder along with general medical issues relevant to cardiovascular disease. Upon completion of these sessions, nurse case managers provided continuous care management by acting as a liaison among patients and existing medical and psychiatric providers. Decision support was implemented through two 1-hour continuing medical education sessions for providers of medical and psychiatric care focused on the unique aspects of cardiovascular risk factors in individuals with bipolar disorder as well as strategies for managing these risk factors based on the American Diabetes Association and American Heart Association guidelines. Pocket cards were also provided to reinforce material in these sessions. Providers in both the intervention and usual care arms of the study had access to the VA's electronic medical record system including records from all care in the VA system. The study intervention did not include elements of enhanced access or community linkages. The study intervention was based largely on Wagner's Chronic Care Model.

Druss and colleagues (2010)[54] conducted a good-quality RCT evaluating medical care management using a registered nurse care manager in an urban community mental health center setting compared to usual care. The nurse care manager functioned not as a member of a team, but rather served as a liaison between medical and mental health providers. Patient self-management skills were supported through motivational interviewing, development of action plans, and coaching to help patients become more active in their own health care. Participants were linked to community resources for child care and public transportation to appointments. The study did not report that access to primary care providers was explicitly enhanced, though system level barriers were addressed by assisting eligible patients to enroll in entitlement programs. The study intervention did not include additional decision support or enhancement of information systems.

Summary of Findings

The four studies represented in our review were similar in many ways, showing a relatively limited variety of approaches to improving general medical care. All studies used nurse care or case managers to some extent to augment or facilitate care provided by physicians or nurse practitioners. Notably, disciplines such as psychologists, with expertise in facilitating behavior change, and nutritionists were not incorporated into the models tested. As described above, three of the four studies had substantial basis in the Chronic Care Model, but elements of PCMH, such as having a primary treating provider, team-based care, and enhanced access, were not robustly employed. Three of the four studies were set in the VA system, while one was a non-VA study.

KEY QUESTION 2. Do models of integrated care for individuals with SMI improve the process of care for preventive services (e.g., colorectal cancer screening) and chronic disease management (e.g., annual eye examination in patients with diabetes mellitus [DM]?

Studies of Efficacy

Two good-quality trials[54,60] provided data relevant to KQ 2. Process of care outcomes are summarized for preventive services (Table 4) and chronic disease management (Table 5). At baseline, the quality of general medical care was low, leaving ample room for intervention effects. In both studies, a high proportion (52 to 54%) of medical diagnoses were not documented previously in the medical record, and in one study,[60] only about 20 percent of recommended preventive services had been provided prior to study start.[54]

In both studies, the intervention improved preventive care as measured by receipt of immunizations and screening tests. Druss and colleagues (2001)[60] reported higher influenza vaccination rates in the intervention versus usual care group (32.2% versus 11.5%, p = 0.006), while more subjects in usual care versus intervention received the pneumococcal vaccination (32.8% versus 11.9%, p = 0.006). This latter difference was not statistically significant in the subgroup with an indication for pneumococcal vaccination.

Selected screening tests were also more likely to be performed in the intervention group than in the usual care group: digital rectal examination (69.5% versus 44.3%, p = 0.005) and flexible sigmoidoscopy (33.9% versus 14.8%, p = 0.01).[60] The investigators also reported a nonsignificant difference favoring the intervention for hemoccult testing (49.2% versus 44.3%, p = 0.10). In the more recent study,[54] a broader set of general medical process measures were evaluated. Immunization outcomes were reported as the proportion of recommended services received (influenza; hepatitis B; measles, mumps, and rubella; pneumococcal; tetanus-diphtheria; and varicella). The intervention group was more likely to receive indicated vaccinations than the usual care group (24.6% versus 3.8%, p < 0.001). In addition, other recommended screening services (cholesterol, fecal occult blood, HIV, sigmoidoscopy, and tuberculosis testing) were completed more frequently in the intervention than usual care group (50.4% versus 21.6%, p < 0.001).[54]

The effects of the intervention on chronic disease management focused on process outcomes relevant to cardiovascular disease risk. Druss and colleagues (2001)[60] reported significantly higher rates in the intervention group for weight measurement, diabetes screening, cholesterol screening, and smoking education. In the intervention group, these services were provided to 71.2 to 84.7% percent of the subjects by study end compared to 45.9 to 63.9 percent in the usual care group. In the later study, [54]Druss and colleagues found higher rates of indicated services for cardiovascular disease (34.9 versus 27.7%, p = 0.03) in the intervention group in an analysis established a priori of a subset of 202 subjects who had one or more cardiometabolic conditions (diabetes, hypertension, hypercholesterolemia, or coronary artery disease). In the subset with blood tests available, the Framingham Cardiac Index (a measure of the 10-year risk of myocardial infarction or coronary-related death) was also significantly lower in the intervention group at study end (6.9 versus 9.8%, p = 0.03), with the intervention group's index improving and the usual care group's index worsening during the course of the study. However, an analysis that adjusted for baseline cardiovascular risk did not show a statistically significant change in risk between groups.

Table 4. Process of care outcomes for preventive care (KQ 2)

Study	Design	Intervention summary	Preventive care			
			Immunizations		Screening procedures	
			Intervention	Control	Intervention	Control
Druss et al., 2001[60] (additional preventive care results reported)	RCT	Co-located general medical clinic with care provided by a nurse practitioner with supervision from a family practitioner. Care coordination provided by a nurse.	• Flu: 32.2% • Pneumovax: 11.9%	• Flu: 11.5% • Pneumovax: 32.8%	• Hemoccult: 49.2% • Digital rectal exam: 65.9% • Flexible sigmoidoscopy: 33.9%	• Hemoccult: 44.3% • Digital rectal exam: 44.3% • Flexible sigmoidoscopy: 14.8%
Druss et al., 2010[54] (additional preventive care results reported)	RCT	Nurse care management with self-management, liaison, and case management components.	Intervention 24.7%[a]	Control 3.8%[a]	Intervention 50.4%[b]	Control 21.6%[b]

[a] Rate reported is percentage of recommended immunizations performed (influenza; hepatitis B; measles, mumps, and rubella; pneumococcal bacterial infection; tetanus-diphtheria; and varicella).
[b] Rate reported is percentage of recommended screening tests performed (cholesterol, fecal blood, HIV, sigmoid, and tuberculosis).
Abbreviation: RCT = randomized controlled trial

Table 5. Process of care outcomes for chronic disease management (KQ 2)

Study	Design	Intervention summary	Chronic disease management	
			Intervention	Control
Druss et al., 2001[60]	RCT	Co-located general medical clinic with care provided by a nurse practitioner with supervision from a family practitioner. Care coordination provided by a nurse.	• (At 12 mo) Diabetes screening: 71.2% • Cholesterol screening: 79.7% • Weight measured?: 84.7% • Smoking education 84.7%	• Diabetes screening: 45.9% • Cholesterol screening: 57.4% • Weight measured: 59.0% • Smoking education: 63.9%
Druss et al., 2010[54]	RCT	Nurse care management with self-management, liaison, and case management components.	• Proportion of indicated services received for cardiovascular disease: 34.9%[a] • Framingham Cardiac Index: 6.9%	• Proportion of indicated services received for cardiovascular disease: 27.7% • Framingham Cardiac Index: 9.8%

[a] Rate reported is the proportion indicated of services received for cardiovascular disease among the subset with at least one cardiometabolic condition (diabetes, hypertension, hypercholesterolemia, or coronary artery disease).
Abbreviation: RCT = randomized controlled trial

Summary of Findings

Only two of the four studies identified for this review reported on measures relevant to KQ 2. Generally, the study interventions improved process measures for preventive services, and cardiovascular disease management. However, some measures represented a "low bar," such as measuring weight rather than evaluating the quality of care for weight control. Other measures of relevant care processes (e.g., physical activity counseling) were not reported. Although rates of recommended services were improved by the intervention, they remained suboptimal in all groups at study end.

KEY QUESTION 3. (3a) Do models of integrated care for individuals with SMI improve general functional status outcomes (e.g., as measured by SF-36) or disease-specific functional status outcomes (e.g., Seattle Angina Questionnaire) related to medical care for chronic medical conditions such as DM, hypertension, or heart failure? (3b) Do models of integrated care for individuals with SMI improve clinical outcomes related to preventive services (e.g., influenza rates) and chronic medical care (e.g., kidney disease, amputations, retinopathy in patients with coexisting DM)?

Studies of Efficacy

Four good-quality studies met our criteria for KQ 3a. All studies measured general functional status outcomes, described in Table 6. Of these, three used the SF-36 item Short-Form Survey[65-67] and one used the SF-12 item Short-Form Survey.[68] Neither disease-specific symptom scales nor disease-specific functional status scales were reported in any of the studies. In addition, none of the four trials met our criteria for KQ3b by reporting clinical outcomes related to preventative services (e.g., incidence of influenza illness) or chronic medical care (e.g., diabetic retinopathy). Brief descriptions of relevant outcomes for each study are described below. Table 7 summarizes outcomes.

Druss and colleagues (2001)[60] reported scores at 52-week followup on the physical health component of the SF-36 Short-Form Survey. Mean scores were higher for the intervention than for usual care group (50.9 [SD 7.1] versus 45.3 [SD 9.7], p = NR). The difference in change between the two groups was significant (t_{170} = 3.7, P<0.001), with subjects in the integrated care clinic scoring 4.7 points higher than baseline in the physical component summary score compared to a 0.3 point decline from baseline in the score of subjects in the general medicine clinic. Higher scores indicated better functional status, and a five-point difference is generally considered a clinically important difference.

Kilbourne and colleagues (2008)[57,59] used the physical health component of the SF-12 Short-Form Survey to report functional outcomes after 24 weeks of the bipolar disorder medical care model versus usual care. The bipolar disorder medical care intervention did not address general medical problems directly but emphasized enrollment in and collaboration with primary care. Change in SF-12 scores from baseline to 24-week follow up differed significantly between intervention and control groups (intervention change in score = 0.8 [SD 6.7] versus control change in score -0.6 [SD 6.6]; p = 0.04).

Investigators in the VA Cooperative Study[55,56,58] as well as Druss and colleagues (2010)[54] also reported on functional outcomes using the SF-36 questionnaire. In the VA Cooperative Study, there was no statistically significant difference at 3-year followup between the Bipolar Collaborative Chronic Care Model and usual care groups on the SF-36 physical health component (mean = 43.4, 95% confidence interval [CI], 42.4 to 44.4 versus mean = 42.9, 95% CI, 41.9 to 43.9). Similarly, Druss and colleagues (2010)[54] did not report a statistically significant difference between the mean scores of intervention versus usual care group on the SF-36 physical health component, although their findings exhibited a trend toward significance. At 1-year followup, SF-36 physical component scores were 37.1 (SD 11.5) and 34.7 (SD 11.9) for the medical care management and usual care groups respectively (p = 0.08). They also noted that the difference in change between the two group scores was not statistically significant (intervention group +1.9% versus usual care group -2.8%). This Druss study was the only one of the four reviewed that focused on an urban community mental health center and did not include veterans.

Table 6. Outcome measures

Measure	General class	Items measured	Scoring range; population mean (SD)	Direction for better outcomes
SF-36	36-item Short Form Health Survey	Physical functioning, role limitations due to physical health problems, bodily pain, general health	0 to 100; 50 (10)	Higher scores indicate better outcomes
SF-12	12-item Short Form Health Survey	Physical functioning, role limitations due to physical health problems, bodily pain, general health	0 to 100; 50 (10)	Higher scores indicate better outcomes

Table 7. Outcome summary for KQ 3

Study	Followup	Intervention versus control outcome
Druss et al., 2001[60]	52 weeks	SF-36 physical component: mean 50.9 (SD 7.1) vs. 45.3 (SD 9.7); p <0.001 for difference in change scores using baseline, 6-month and 12-month assessments
Bauer et al., 2006[55,56] Kilbourne et al., 2009[58] (VA Cooperative Study)	156 weeks	SF-36 physical component: mean 43.4 (95% CI, 42.4 to 44.4) vs. 42.9 (95% CI, 41.9 to 43.9)
Kilbourne et al., 2008[57,59]	12 weeks 24 weeks	SF-12 physical component: mean 38.5 (SD 8.4) vs. 33.9 (SD 8.6), p = NR SF-12 physical component: mean 37.0 (SD 7.3) vs. 35.1 (SD 7.7), p = NR; difference in change scores using baseline, 3 month and 6 month assessments: 2.5, 95% CI, 0.5 to 4.9
Druss et al., 2010[54]	52 weeks	SF-36 physical component: mean 37.1 (SD 11.5) versus 34.7 (SD 11.9); p < 0.08; difference in change scores: "not significant," p value not reported

Abbreviation: CI = confidence interval; NR = not reported; p = probability; SD = standard deviation; SF = Short Form

Summary of Findings

In summary, the findings from two good-quality RCTs provided support for small improvements in general functional outcomes at followup periods ranging up to 52 weeks. Two other RCTs did not find statistically significant differences using similar health outcome survey measures when comparing integrated care to usual care. Thus, effects on physical function appear small and inconsistent. However, interventions varied in their focus on care processes that could be expected to improve physical function. Followup periods ranged from 24 to 156 weeks, and interventions that focus primarily on preventive care could be expected to require long followup periods to show positive effects on physical functioning. Three of the four studies were conducted in the VA system, with two of three VA studies demonstrating improvements in general functional outcomes. Given the range of medical services generally offered on site at VA health care locations, integration and collocation approaches may be easier to implement, and VA interventions generalize more easily to VA settings.

We did not identify published trials or quasi-experimental studies examining clinical outcomes relating to preventative services.

KEY QUESTION 4. What are the gaps in evidence for determining how best to integrate care to improve general medical outcomes for individuals with SMI?

Only four trials, comprising 891 individuals, were identified by this review. The relatively small number of trials and limited range of outcomes reported make definitive conclusions difficult. Further, the small number of trials makes it difficult to identify the key elements of the interventions. We summarize the gaps in evidence in Table 8 and then discuss these gaps further.

Table 8. Summary of gaps in evidence

The key intervention components are uncertain.
There is greater uncertainty about intervention effects for individuals with SMIs other than bipolar disorder.
Effects on clinical outcomes have not been studied.
Sustainability of intervention effects is uncertain.
Effects of interventions (effectiveness) are uncertain when part of routine care rather than part of an RCT.
Effects of current VA delivery models are uncertain, including primary care services co-located in the mental health setting and assertive community treatment.
There is uncertainty about effects of current VA programs to improve mental health outcomes of veterans with SMI (e.g., assertive community treatment) that theoretically may have beneficial effects on general medical outcomes.

Abbreviation: RCT = randomized controlled trial; SMI = serious mental illness; VA = Veterans Affairs

The four RCTs included in our review, as reported in KQ 1, offered interventions with multiple components—with all components offered to those receiving the intervention. These study designs did not permit disaggregation of intervention effects for each intervention component.

Because two studies focused entirely on individuals with bipolar disorder, the proportion of studies with other SMIs was relatively few, with just 19 percent of the overall samples identified as having schizophrenia or schizoaffective disorder. The two studies that included individuals with SMI other than bipolar disorder did not provide subgroup analyses by diagnosis, so possible differences in the efficacy of the study interventions between diagnostic groups is unknown. Global Assessment of Functioning was reported in only one trial and only by study assignment group, so it was not possible to determine the overall number of individuals who met our study criteria based on level of functioning.

None of the four trials provided information on general medical outcomes, such as rates of diabetic neuropathy, influenza, or myocardial infarction, that occurred in study populations either during the delivery of the study intervention or in follow-up. While many measures selected for process of preventive care and quality of chronic disease management are known to be correlated with clinical outcomes, absence of this information is a substantial gap in the evidence. It may be possible, particularly for the three studies conducted in VA settings, to obtain additional follow-up data on general medical outcomes on study subjects.

Three of the four studies[54,57,60] evaluated interventions implemented at only one site. Only one study[60] explicitly stated that existing staff or resources were used in the study intervention, with the other trials delivering interventions with staff funded with research grants. Therefore, the RCTs reviewed primarily provided evidence regarding efficacy of the study interventions under ideal and closely controlled conditions. Information about the effectiveness of these interventions when implemented in existing programs was lacking.

All of the studies included in this review were RCTs with randomization at the patient level. No studies were identified using other designs stated in our inclusion criteria, such as cluster randomized trials, nonrandomized cluster controlled trials, controlled before-and-after studies, or interrupted time series designs. These additional designs can yield different types of information from the patient-level RCT, given that they are most often conducted in natural environments, thus producing fewer threats to external validity. For example, three of the four RCTs were conducted in single sites where motivation of the researchers and clinicians was likely to be high. Multisite designs might provide broader information on the effectiveness of the interventions in more naturalistic settings.

Two models of delivery of care that have already been implemented in the VA are relevant to our study questions: programs with co-located mental health and primary care and assertive community treatment programs. Mental health–primary care programs, which serve veterans with SMI in a clinic organized under the mental health service and are often co-located with mental health clinics, have been implemented in 10 out of 107 VA medical centers, based on a national survey of mental health leaders. After adjustment for organizational and patient-level factors, analyses of data from these programs showed that patients from co-located clinics received better quality of care compared with those without co-location on four of nine indicators. The study showed a need for additional chronic disease management strategies in these co-located clinics, given that HgA1c was actually less well controlled in these clinics compared to those without co-location. Another study using VA data in these co-located clinics, compared to those without co-location, showed a significant reduction in hospitalizations for ambulatory care–sensitive conditions.[69,70] Additional evaluation of these programs, even retrospectively, has the potential to provide valuable information relevant to our study questions, including filling some of the gaps in evidence identified here (e.g., lack of quasi-experimental designs, broader diversity of included subjects based on diagnosis, and reporting of general medical outcomes).

Assertive community treatment—implemented in the VA as Mental Health Intensive Case Management (MHICM)—has been shown to be effective in reducing symptom severity and inpatient psychiatric utilization among individuals with SMI; client-reported housing, quality of life, satisfaction with services are improved.[71] Though these programs, and their evaluation, to date have been focused on mental health outcomes, case managers do facilitate receipt of primary care services to varying degrees—yet general medical outcomes of patients receiving MHICM and other assertive community treatment implementations have been largely unreported.

It is notable that the collaborative care models for bipolar disorder employed in two of the studies [55,57] have gained sufficient evidence to be included in the recommendations of two recent clinical treatment guidelines.[72,73] Still, the impact of these models on general medical outcomes remains an area where additional study is needed.

Our search of www.clinicaltrials.gov identified three RCTs and one observational study evaluating integrated approaches to addressing the general medical needs of individuals with SMI. One of these studies is being conducted in VHA. These studies are summarized in Table 9.

Table 9. Ongoing studies evaluating integrated approaches

Study title	VA/DOD population?	Intervention	Comparator	Sponsor and ClinicalTrials.gov ID number	Funding start and stop date	Status
Life Goals Behavioral Change to Improve Outcomes for Veterans With Serious Mental Illness	Y	Behavioral: life goals collaborative care	Usual care	Department of Veterans Affairs NCT01244854	October 2010 to December 2011	Enrolling by invitation
Treatment of Metabolic Syndrome in a Community Mental Health Center	N	IMBED: active comparator—a primary care provider Liaison: Active comparator—a medical case manager	Treatment as usual; no intervention	The University of Texas Health Science Center at San Antonio NCT01115114	January 2009 to September 2012	Recruiting
The Medical HOME Study	N	Care team	No intervention; referral only	National Institute of Mental Health NCT01228032	April 2010 to January 2015	Recruiting
Non-RCT						
Reduction of Cardiovascular Risk in Severe Mental Illness (RISCA-TMS)	N	Nurse-administered lifestyle counseling	None	Consorci Hospitalari de Vic NCT01182012	August 2010 to December 2012	Recruiting
Benefits of a Primary Care Clinic Co-located and Integrated in the Mental Health Setting for Veterans with Serious Mental Illness	Y	Enrollment in a co-located, integrated primary care clinic in the mental health outpatient unit	Subject is own comparator; time-series design	Systems Outcomes and Quality in Chronic Disease and Rehabilitation; Providence VA Medical Center	Unfunded	Completed; manuscript in press

Abbreviations: RCT = randomized controlled trial

SUMMARY AND DISCUSSION

A key observation that emerges from this review is that integration of care for the purpose of improving general medical outcomes in individuals with SMI is an understudied area, with only four RCTs meeting our study criteria. Further, these studies tested a limited range of approaches to integrating care. Despite these limitations, these four studies provided useful findings for several of our key questions. These findings and the overall strength of evidence are summarized and discussed by key question.

SUMMARY OF EVIDENCE BY KEY QUESTION

Table 10. Strength of evidence by key question

Key question	Strength of evidence	Summary
KQ 1. What types of care models have been evaluated prospectively that integrate mental health care and primary medical care with the goal of improving general medical outcomes for individuals with serious mental illness (SMI)?	Not relevant to KQ 1	4 good-quality studies Conclusions: • The degree of integration of care ranged from limited to moderate. • The range of integrated care models tested was relatively limited. Many PCMH elements were not included in tested models. • A broader range of disciplines should be included in future evaluations of integrated care models.
KQ 2. Do models of integrated care for individuals with SMI improve the process of care for preventive services (e.g., colorectal cancer screening) and chronic disease management (e.g., annual eye examination in patients with diabetes mellitus [DM])?	Moderate	2 good-quality studies Conclusions: • Studies showed generally positive effects on immunization rates, cancer screening, and selected screening for cardiovascular disease. • Important cancer-screening practices (e.g., mammography, pap smears) and chronic disease care unrelated to cardiovascular disease were not studied.
KQ 3. (3a) Do models of integrated care for individuals with SMI improve general functional status outcomes (e.g., as measured by SF-36) or disease-specific functional status outcomes (e.g., Seattle Angina Questionnaire) related to medical care for chronic medical conditions such as DM, hypertension, or heart failure? (3b) Do models of integrated care for individuals with SMI improve clinical outcomes related to preventive services (e.g., influenza rates) and chronic medical care (e.g., kidney disease, amputations, retinopathy in patients with coexisting DM)?	Moderate for KQ 3a Insufficient for KQ 3b	4 good-quality studies for KQ 3a; no studies reported data relevant to KQ 3b Conclusions: • Studies reported inconsistent effects on physical functional status. Two studies showed small, positive effects, and two showed no statistically or clinically significant benefit. • No study reported effects on disease-specific functional status or clinical outcomes.

Key question	Strength of evidence	Summary
KQ 4. What are the gaps in evidence for determining how best to integrate care to improve general medical outcomes for individuals with SMI?	Not relevant to KQ 4	4 good-quality studies Conclusions: • There was little diversity in the types of models tested, with most models based on Wagner's Chronic Care Model. • Elements of PCMH, other than those that overlap with the chronic care model, were not generally evaluated. • Other than cardiovascular disease, greater variety of chronic disease outcomes is missing in the literature. • There was relatively little evidence regarding individuals with schizophrenia and related psychotic disorders.

Abbreviation: DM = diabetes mellitus; KQ = key question; PCMH = patient-centered medical home; SF = Short Form; SMI = serious mental illness

KQ 1

For KQ 1, four RCTs (represented by seven articles) evaluated approaches to integrated care and most commonly were theoretically based on the chronic care model. All integrated care models were set in mental health specialty settings, had additional personnel, and used care management or care coordination as a key strategy. Only one study used co-located mental health and general medical services. Self-management support was a component in three of the four studies, but only one study used decision support for general medical care.

Within VHA, general medical and psychiatric services are most often provided in settings that are organizationally and geographically distinct. Integrating these services for patients with SMI has the potential to improve outcomes. At the simplest level, the integration of mental and physical health care takes place when specialty mental health and general medical providers collaborate to address the mental and physical health needs of their patients. Broadly speaking, integration can occur in two ways: specialty mental health care being introduced into general medical settings or general medical care being introduced into specialty mental health settings. A robust literature shows that integrating mental health services into primary care improves mental health outcomes. In contrast, few trials have tested approaches to integrating care to improve general medical outcomes for patients with SMI. On the spectrum of limited integration (e.g., communication between providers) to fully integrated (e.g., shared development and implementation of the treatment plan), the interventions tested range from limited[55,56,58] to moderately integrated.[60]

Although these interventions have been informed by the chronic care model, elements such as decision support, shared decisionmaking, self-management support related to chronic medical conditions, and community linkages have not been commonly included. If the conceptual model were broadened to include elements of PCMH, then additional elements such as designated care teams, shared medical appointments, home telemonitoring, test and referral tracking, and performance monitoring might be tested. Implementing the PCMH in VHA—known as the Patient Aligned Care Team (PACT)—provides a potential opportunity to test these models for individuals with SMI. The locus of care for such a model for individuals with SMI is yet to be determined. The studies identified maintained mental health settings as the central point of care with services either augmented in these settings by co-located general medical services, or by placing care managers in the mental health setting to facilitate care in the general medical setting. Given the intensity of psychiatric services often required and provided in this population, this may be a logical approach; however, studies where psychiatric services were provided to augment general medical services in the general medical setting were not identified. It is possible that the general medical and mental health needs of some individuals with SMI can be adequately provided within the context of PACT, but this model of care has not yet been formally evaluated. Finally, by emphasizing the team-care approach essential to PACT, these models could test multidisciplinary teams that include nutritionists and psychologists or health educators to address needed behavior changes. Consistent with the transformation of VA mental health services towards a recovery orientation, peer support interventions may also be useful, with one pilot study showing benefit for patient activation and number of primary care visits in a study of veterans with SMI.[74]

Another potential strategy that does not appear to have been studied is the training of mental health professionals to directly manage some common general medical illnesses. It is possible that this strategy could improve general medical outcomes in individuals with SMI without increasing the burden on primary care services. However, interventions that attempt to improve mental health care through training primary care providers have been largely ineffective.

KQ 2

Two good-quality trials involving 527 patients reported outcomes relevant to KQ 2. These studies showed generally positive effects on immunization rates, cancer screening, and selected screening for cardiovascular disease. We rated the strength of evidence for these outcomes as moderate. However, important cancer-screening practices (e.g., mammography, pap smears) and chronic disease care unrelated to cardiovascular disease were not studied.

When examined in detail, these studies showed important differences in intervention design, with Druss and colleagues (2001)[60] co-locating primary care services in the mental health setting in a VA medical center and Druss and colleagues (2010)[54] providing care management in an urban community mental health center to facilitate care with various primary care providers in the community. In the later study, primary care providers were organizationally and physically separate from the community mental health center. These studies provide evidence that integrated care models can improve preventive services and chronic disease management as compared with usual care—one in an integrated system and one in a nonintegrated system. Both studies included a broad range of individuals with SMI. Given the theoretical reasons, as shown in our analytic framework, for differential effects by specific mental illnesses, social support systems, and severity of chronic medical illnesses, larger studies in multiple sites would be helpful to further understand the impact of integrated care models on these outcomes for individuals with SMI.

KQ 3

For KQ 3, four good-quality trials reported inconsistent effects on physical components of functional status. Two studies showed small, positive effects, and two showed no statistically or clinically significant benefit. We rated the strength of evidence for the finding of no to small positive effects on physical functioning as "moderate." No study reported disease-specific functional status or clinical outcomes. We rated the strength of evidence "insufficient" for these outcomes.

Integrated care models, ranging from limited to moderate levels of integration, had inconsistent effects on the physical component of functional status for individuals with SMI. Additional studies may help to clarify these mixed results. Interventions that are more tailored to specific disease states, or utilize greater levels of integration and organizational support may be required to produce more robust effects on functional status. That there were no studies providing data on clinical outcomes, such as disease-specific or all-cause mortality rates, is a significant gap in the literature. However, numerous studies among the general population have demonstrated strong links between process measures for prevention and chronic disease management and improvement in clinical outcomes. Given the size and duration of studies required to demonstrate differences in ultimate clinical outcomes for these issues, studies that assess well-established intermediate outcomes may be adequate, particularly given potentially higher priority gaps in the literature. In addition, there is not a strong reason to believe that process outcome linkages would differ for the general and SMI populations. However, incorporation of disease-specific symptom and physical function measures would be feasible and should be strongly considered in future trials.

KQ 4

Among the four studies reviewed, there was relatively little diversity in the types of models tested, with most models based on Wagner's Chronic Care Model. Elements of PCMH, other than those that overlap with the chronic care model, were not generally evaluated. Other models, including community-based care approaches may hold promise but were not evaluated in this review. At this early stage in the development of interventions to improve general medical outcomes, researchers and policymakers should remain open to alternative models.

With cardiovascular disease being a main source of morbidity and mortality in the general population and particularly in individuals with SMI, the focus on this category of disease is important. However, a greater variety of chronic disease outcomes is missing in the literature. Finally, there was relatively little evidence regarding individuals with schizophrenia and related psychotic disorders.

Important gaps in the literature were identified in our review. These gaps are further discussed in the Recommendations for Future Research section below.

LIMITATIONS

The term "serious mental illness" varies in definition—an issue that makes it challenging to study this population through systematic reviews. Serious mental illness is not a MeSH search term, making searches of electronic databases challenging. Although we used broad and sensitive search strategies across multiple databases and augmented the searches by reviewing the bibliographies of selected articles, our search strategy may still have missed relevant articles. Three of the four studies were conducted in VA settings, possibly limiting applicability outside of nonintegrated health care systems.

In addition to the above limitations, our methodological approach had important strengths. First, limiting our review to evidence gleaned from clinical trials and quasi-experimental studies allowed us to focus on quality over quantity when examining this relatively undeveloped body of research. In addition, our evidence synthesis was guided by a carefully designed standardized protocol, including a systematic search of research databases and relevant bibliographies, double data abstraction, and use of validated criteria to assess the quality of identified studies. Further, we searched for evidence of publication bias in ClinicalTrials.gov. In sum, this was a highly structured and systematic review of the extant evidence.

RECOMMENDATIONS FOR FUTURE RESEARCH

The combination of the known gaps in the quality of general medical care and subsequent outcomes in this population, together with the few relevant studies identified, confirms the importance of future research in this area. Proven interventions that close gaps in quality and can be implemented widely are needed. The ultimate goal is to improve general medical outcomes for individuals with serious mental illnesses; however none of the studies identified reports distal clinical outcomes, such as disease-specific symptom measures or disease-specific or all-cause mortality rates. Future research should include longer-term follow up and patient important clinical outcomes, particularly in the absence of a strong process – outcome association for intermediate outcomes.

SMIs encompass a wide variety of psychopathologies. Individuals with various psychiatric diagnoses within this broad group may, by virtue of the nature of their psychiatric symptoms, have differences in their experience of general medical care, leading to disparate outcomes among these subgroups. Individuals with bipolar disorder comprised two of the four studies identified here. A considerable amount of research has been conducted in the VHA and elsewhere that demonstrates significant disparities in outcomes and quality measures for individuals with other disorders, including and perhaps especially, schizophrenia and related disorders. Yet, studies here included a relatively small number of individuals with these disorders identified, with no analyses conducted by subgroup. While some methods to improve integration of care for individuals with SMI may be generalized among these diagnostic entities, some may need to be more specific to the psychiatric diagnostic group. Future research could focus on integration of psychiatric and general medical care for individuals with schizophrenia and related disorders as well as other diagnostic subgroups.

With the exception of the study by Bauer and colleagues (2006),[55,56,58] all of the identified studies were conducted in one site, and all of the studies identified used clinical staff funded through research studies. Larger studies in more naturalistic, real-world settings are needed to evaluate the effectiveness, as opposed to efficacy, of the strategies tested. The models used in the studies in this review could be described broadly as:

1. Co-location of primary care services in the mental health setting.[60]
2. Optimization of treatment for psychiatric illness through collaborative care in the mental health setting with enhanced enrollment in and collaboration with primary care.[55,56,58]
3. Modification of the collaborative care model for psychiatric illness to specifically address common general medical issues seen in individuals with SMI.[57,59]

4. Nurse care management, focused on general medical issues, provided in the mental health setting to increase information exchange, access to primary care, and collaboration with primary care providers.[54]

The VA Cooperative Studies Program provides an valuable infrastructure for testing the effectiveness of larger scale implementation of these models, perhaps using RCTs with randomization at the site level. A large multicenter study might also allow for disaggregation of effects of various model components.

While our systematic review intentionally excluded interventions delivered in the community, the mental health outcomes associated with assertive community treatment emphasize the effectiveness of community-based interventions in this population. Assertive community treatment, implemented in the VA as Mental Health Intensive Case Management, operates under multiple principles, including that most services are provided within the team as opposed to being brokered out to other providers. The inclusion of a primary care provider, integrated into the workings of an assertive community treatment team, has not been studied as a platform for delivery of primary care services to this population. The model used in Druss and colleagues (2010)[54] could be applied to the assertive community treatment model, with case managers having increased emphasis on coordination of services for general medical illnesses and disease registries implemented to assure preventive services are delivered. While we limited studies in this review to those conducted in traditional mental health outpatient settings, services delivered in the community may also be important to improving general medical care in this population.

Additional sites of delivery of mental health services focusing on individuals with SMI could potentially be targets for studying the addition of services oriented toward general physical health. For example, in the VA, Psychosocial Rehabilitation and Recovery Centers (PRRCs) provide treatment and rehabilitation services to Veterans with SMI. The addition of primary care services and the impact of wellness-oriented activities could be studied in PRRCs. Also, some VA Community Based Outpatient Centers (CBOCs) have developed integrated care programs. There may be a ready opportunity to conduct a high-quality observational study comparing these centers to CBOCs without integrated care programs.

By design, our review did not address disparities in quality of care received by individuals with SMI in general medical inpatient settings. Gaps in quality of care may also exist in inpatient care received by individuals with SMI, as has been shown for myocardial infarction[32] and in receipt of and outcomes after nonemergency surgical procedures.[75] These issues were beyond the scope of the current review but may be important topics for future systematic reviews.

REFERENCES

1. Chang C-K, Hayes R, Broadbent M, et al. All-cause mortality among people with serious mental illness (SMI), substance use disorders, and depressive disorders in southeast London: a cohort study. *BMC Psychiatry*. 2010;10(1):77.

2. Brown AS, Birthwhistle J. Excess mortality of mental illness. *Br J Psychiatry*. 1996;169(3):383-4.

3. Parks J, Svendsen D, Singer P, et al. Morbidity and Mortality in People with Serious Mental Illness (Technical Report 13). Alexandria, VA: National Association of State Mental Health Progaram Directors. 2006.

4. Colton CW, Manderscheid RW. Congruencies in increased mortality rates, years of potential life lost, and causes of death among public mental health clients in eight states. *Prev Chronic Dis*. 2006;3(2):A42.

5. Hennekens CH. Increasing global burden of cardiovascular disease in general populations and patients with schizophrenia. *J Clin Psychiatry*. 2007;68 Suppl 4:4-7.

6. Kilbourne AM, Morden NE, Austin K, et al. Excess heart-disease-related mortality in a national study of patients with mental disorders: identifying modifiable risk factors. *Gen Hosp Psychiatry*. 2009;31(6):555-63.

7. Wu EQ, Birnbaum HG, Shi L, et al. The economic burden of schizophrenia in the United States in 2002. *J Clin Psychiatry*. 2005;66(9):1122-9.

8. Peele PB, Xu Y, Kupfer DJ. Insurance expenditures on bipolar disorder: clinical and parity implications. *Am J Psychiatry*. 2003;160(7):1286-90.

9. Merikangas KR, Akiskal HS, Angst J, et al. Lifetime and 12-month prevalence of bipolar spectrum disorder in the National Comorbidity Survey replication. *Arch Gen Psychiatry*. 2007;64(5):543-52.

10. Simon GE, Unutzer J. Health care utilization and costs among patients treated for bipolar disorder in an insured population. *Psychiatr Serv*. 1999;50(10):1303-8.

11. Bryant-Comstock L, Stender M, Devercelli G. Health care utilization and costs among privately insured patients with bipolar I disorder. *Bipolar Disord*. 2002;4(6):398-405.

12. Rosenberg SD, Swanson JW, Wolford GL, et al. The five-site health and risk study of blood-borne infections among persons with severe mental illness. *Psychiatr Serv*. 2003;54(6):827-35.

13. Hsu JH, Chien IC, Lin CH, et al. Incidence of diabetes in patients with schizophrenia: a population-based study. *Can J Psychiatry*. 2011;56(1):19-26.

14. Dixon L, Weiden P, Delahanty J, et al. Prevalence and correlates of diabetes in national schizophrenia samples. *Schizophr Bull*. 2000;26(4):903-12.

15. van Winkel R, De Hert M, Van Eyck D, et al. Prevalence of diabetes and the metabolic syndrome in a sample of patients with bipolar disorder. *Bipolar Disord*. 2008;10(2):342-8.

16. Sokal J, Messias E, Dickerson FB, et al. Comorbidity of medical illnesses among adults with serious mental illness who are receiving community psychiatric services. *J Nerv Ment Dis*. 2004;192(6):421-7.

17. Bresee LC, Majumdar SR, Patten SB, et al. Prevalence of cardiovascular risk factors and disease in people with schizophrenia: a population-based study. *Schizophr Res*. 2010;117(1):75-82.

18. Weiner M, Warren L, Fiedorowicz JG. Cardiovascular morbidity and mortality in bipolar disorder. *Ann Clin Psychiatry*. 2011;23(1):40-7.

19. McCreadie RG. Diet, smoking and cardiovascular risk in people with schizophrenia: descriptive study. *Br J Psychiatry*. 2003;183:534-9.

20. McElroy SL. Obesity in patients with severe mental illness: overview and management. *J Clin Psychiatry*. 2009;70 Suppl 3:12-21.

21. Fountoulakis KN, Siamouli M, Panagiotidis P, et al. Obesity and smoking in patients with schizophrenia and normal controls: a case-control study. *Psychiatry Res*. 2010;176(1):13-6.

22. Swartz MS, Wagner HR, Swanson JW, et al. Substance Use and Psychosocial Functioning in Schizophrenia Among New Enrollees in the NIMH CATIE Study. *Psychiatr Serv*. 2006;57(8):1110-1116.

23. Brown S, Birtwistle J, Roe L, et al. The unhealthy lifestyle of people with schizophrenia. *Psychol Med*. 1999;29(3):697-701.

24. Cohen CI. Poverty and the course of schizophrenia: implications for research and policy. *Hosp Community Psychiatry*. 1993;44(10):951-8.

25. Fischer PJ, Breakey WR. The epidemiology of alcohol, drug, and mental disorders among homeless persons. *Am Psychol*. 1991;46(11):1115-28.

26. Trauer T, Duckmanton RA, Chiu E. A study of the quality of life of the severely mentally ill. *Int J Soc Psychiatry*. 1998;44(2):79-91.

27. Desai MM, Rosenheck RA, Druss BG, et al. Receipt of nutrition and exercise counseling among medical outpatients with psychiatric and substance use disorders. *J Gen Intern Med*. 2002;17(7):556-60.

28. Druss BG, Rosenheck RA, Desai MM, et al. Quality of preventive medical care for patients with mental disorders. *Med Care*. 2002;40(2):129-36.

29. Green JL, Gazmararian JA, Rask KJ, et al. Quality of diabetes care for underserved patients with and without mental illness: site of care matters. *Psychiatr Serv.* 2010;61(12):1204-10.

30. Frayne SM, Halanych JH, Miller DR, et al. Disparities in diabetes care: impact of mental illness. *Arch Intern Med.* 2005;165(22):2631-8.

31. Mitchell AJ, Lord O. Do deficits in cardiac care influence high mortality rates in schizophrenia? A systematic review and pooled analysis. *J Psychopharmacol.* 2010;24(4 Suppl):69-80.

32. Druss BG, Bradford DW, Rosenheck RA, et al. Mental disorders and use of cardiovascular procedures after myocardial infarction. *JAMA.* 2000;283(4):506-11.

33. Ray WA, Chung CP, Murray KT, et al. Atypical antipsychotic drugs and the risk of sudden cardiac death. *N Engl J Med.* 2009;360(3):225-35.

34. Bergman RN, Ader M. Atypical antipsychotics and glucose homeostasis. *J Clin Psychiatry.* 2005;66(4):504-14.

35. Koro CE, Meyer JM. Atypical antipsychotic therapy and hyperlipidemia: a review. *Essent Psychopharmacol.* 2005;6(3):148-57.

36. Wirshing DA. Schizophrenia and obesity: impact of antipsychotic medications. *J Clin Psychiatry.* 2004;65 Suppl 18:13-26.

37. American Board of Internal Medicine. Combined Training Internal Medicine. Available at: www.abim.org/certification/policies/combinedim/compsych.aspx. Accessed June 28, 2011.

38. Druss BG. Improving medical care for persons with serious mental illness: challenges and solutions. *J Clin Psychiatry.* 2007;68 Suppl 4:40-4.

39. Bradford DW, Kim MM, Braxton LE, et al. Access to medical care among persons with psychotic and major affective disorders. *Psychiatr Serv.* 2008;59(8):847-52.

40. Rollman BL, Belnap BH, Mazumdar S, et al. A randomized trial to improve the quality of treatment for panic and generalized anxiety disorders in primary care. *Arch Gen Psychiatry.* 2005;62(12):1332-41.

41. Roy-Byrne P, Craske MG, Sullivan G, et al. Delivery of evidence-based treatment for multiple anxiety disorders in primary care: a randomized controlled trial. *JAMA.* 2010;303(19):1921-8.

42. Butler M, Kane RL, McAlpine D, et al. Integration of mental health/substance abuse and primary care. *Evid Rep Technol Assess (Full Rep).* 2008(173):1-362.

43. Rubenstein LV, Williams JW, Jr., Danz M, et al. Determining Key Features of Effective Depression Interventions. Available at: http://www.ncbi.nlm.nih.gov/books/NBK48533/. Accessed June 28, 2011. 2009.

44. Grumbach K, Bodenheimer T. A primary care home for Americans: putting the house in order. *JAMA*. 2002;288(7):889-93.

45. Stange KC, Nutting PA, Miller WL, et al. Defining and measuring the patient-centered medical home. *J Gen Intern Med*. 2010;25(6):601-12.

46. Gelberg L, Andersen RM, Leake BD. The Behavioral Model for Vulnerable Populations: application to medical care use and outcomes for homeless people. *Health Serv Res*. 2000;34(6):1273-302.

47. Wilczynski NL, Haynes RB, Lavis JN, et al. Optimal search strategies for detecting health services research studies in MEDLINE. *CMAJ*. 2004;171(10):1179-85.

48. Haynes RB, McKibbon KA, Wilczynski NL, et al. Optimal search strategies for retrieving scientifically strong studies of treatment from Medline: analytical survey. *BMJ*. 2005;330(7501):1179.

49. Cochrane Collaboration. Cochrane Handbook for Systematic Reviews of Interventions. Chapter 6: Searching for studies. Section 6.4.11.1, March 2011.

50. Cochrane Effective Practice and Organisation of Care Group. EPOC resources for review authors. Available at: http://epoc.cochrane.org/epoc-resources-review-authors. Accessed June 28, 2011.

51. Bodenheimer T, Wagner EH, Grumbach K. Improving primary care for patients with chronic illness: the chronic care model, Part 2. *JAMA*. 2002;288(15):1909-14.

52. Agency for Healthcare Research and Quality. Methods Guide for Effectiveness and Comparative Effectiveness Reviews. Rockville, MD: Agency for Healthcare Research and Quality. Available at: http://www.effectivehealthcare.ahrq.gov/index.cfm/search-for-guides-reviews-and-reports/?pageaction=displayproduct&productid=318. Accessed June 28, 2011.

53. Guyatt GH, Oxman AD, Vist GE, et al. GRADE: an emerging consensus on rating quality of evidence and strength of recommendations. *BMJ*. 2008;336(7650):924-6.

54. Druss BG, von Esenwein SA, Compton MT, et al. A randomized trial of medical care management for community mental health settings: the Primary Care Access, Referral, and Evaluation (PCARE) study. *Am J Psychiatry*. 2010;167(2):151-9.

55. Bauer MS, McBride L, Williford WO, et al. Collaborative care for bipolar disorder: part I. Intervention and implementation in a randomized effectiveness trial. *Psychiatr Serv*. 2006;57(7):927-36.

56. Bauer MS, McBride L, Williford WO, et al. Collaborative care for bipolar disorder: Part II. Impact on clinical outcome, function, and costs. *Psychiatr Serv*. 2006;57(7):937-45.

57. Kilbourne AM, Post EP, Nossek A, et al. Improving medical and psychiatric outcomes among individuals with bipolar disorder: a randomized controlled trial. *Psychiatr Serv*. 2008;59(7):760-8.

58. Kilbourne AM, Biswas K, Pirraglia PA, et al. Is the collaborative chronic care model effective for patients with bipolar disorder and co-occurring conditions? *J Affect Disord.* 2009;112(1-3):256-61.

59. Kilbourne AM, Post EP, Nossek A, et al. Service delivery in older patients with bipolar disorder: a review and development of a medical care model. *Bipolar Disord.* 2008;10(6):672-83.

60. Druss BG, Rohrbaugh RM, Levinson CM, et al. Integrated medical care for patients with serious psychiatric illness: a randomized trial. *Arch Gen Psychiatry.* 2001;58(9):861-8.

61. Health care reform for Americans with severe mental illnesses: report of the National Advisory Mental Health Council. *Am J Psychiatry.* 1993;150(10):1447-65.

62. Wagner EH. The role of patient care teams in chronic disease management. *BMJ.* 2000;320(7234):569-72.

63. Von Korff M, Gruman J, Schaefer J, et al. Collaborative management of chronic illness. *Ann Intern Med.* 1997;127(12):1097-102.

64. Bodenheimer T, Wagner EH, Grumbach K. Improving primary care for patients with chronic illness. *JAMA.* 2002;288(14):1775-9.

65. Ware JE, Jr., Sherbourne CD. The MOS 36-item short-form health survey (SF-36). I. Conceptual framework and item selection. *Med Care.* 1992;30(6):473-83.

66. McHorney CA, Ware JE, Jr., Raczek AE. The MOS 36-Item Short-Form Health Survey (SF-36): II. Psychometric and clinical tests of validity in measuring physical and mental health constructs. *Med Care.* 1993;31(3):247-63.

67. McHorney CA, Ware JE, Jr., Lu JF, et al. The MOS 36-item Short-Form Health Survey (SF-36): III. Tests of data quality, scaling assumptions, and reliability across diverse patient groups. *Med Care.* 1994;32(1):40-66.

68. Ware J, Jr., Kosinski M, Keller SD. A 12-Item Short-Form Health Survey: construction of scales and preliminary tests of reliability and validity. *Med Care.* 1996;34(3):220-33.

69. Kilbourne AM, Pirraglia PA, Zongshan L, et al. Quality of General Medical Care Among Patients With Serious Mental Illness: Does Colocation of Services Matter? *Psychiatr Serv.* 2011;In press.

70. Pirraglia PA, Kilbourne AM, Lai Z, et al. Colocated general medical care and preventable hospital admissions for veterans with serious mental illness. *Psychiatr Serv.* 2011;62(5):554-7.

71. Rosenheck RA, Neale MS. Cost-effectiveness of intensive psychiatric community care for high users of inpatient services. *Arch Gen Psychiatry.* 1998;55(5):459-66.

72. The Management of Bipolar Disorder Working Group. VA/DoD clinical practice guideline for management of bipolar disorder in adults. Washington (DC): Department of Veterans Affairs, Department of Defense; 2010. Available at: http://www.guideline.gov/content.aspx?id=16314. Accessed August 30, 2011.

73. Yatham LN, Kennedy SH, O'Donovan C, et al. Canadian Network for Mood and Anxiety Treatments (CANMAT) guidelines for the management of patients with bipolar disorder: update 2007. *Bipolar Disord*. 2006;8(6):721-39.

74. Druss BG, Zhao L, von Esenwein SA, et al. The Health and Recovery Peer (HARP) Program: A peer-led intervention to improve medical self-management for persons with serious mental illness. *Schizophr Res*. 2010.

75. Li Y, Cai X, Du H, et al. Mentally ill medicare patients less likely than others to receive certain types of surgery. *Health Aff (Millwood)*. 2011;30(7):1307-15.

APPENDIX A. SEARCH STRATEGY

Step	Category	Terms	Result
1	Eligible disorders	("Serious mental illness") [all fields] OR ("severe mental illness") [all fields] OR schizophrenia [tiab] OR schizophrenia [mesh] OR bipolar disorder [mesh:noexp] OR bipolar disorder [tiab] OR psychotic disorders [mesh:noexp] OR psychotic disorders [tiab] OR schizoaffective disorder* [tiab] OR mania [tiab] OR manic [tiab] OR bipolar affective disorder [tiab] OR *mental disorders [tiab]	790929
2	Interventions	Delivery of Health Care, Integrated [Mesh] OR Patient Care Team [Mesh] OR Patient Care Planning [Mesh] OR Disease Management [Mesh] OR Comprehensive Health Care [Mesh:noexp] OR Patient Care Management [Mesh:noexp] OR Primary Health Care [Mesh] OR Internal Medicine [Mesh] OR Family practice [Mesh] OR Geriatrics [Mesh] OR "general practice" [ti] OR ("continuity of care" OR "coordinated care" OR "coordinated program*" OR "team care" OR "team treatment" OR "team assessment" OR "team consultation") OR (collaborat*[ti] AND care [ti]) OR "shared care" [ti] OR (collaborat*[ti] AND manage*[ti])	292051
3	Study designs	("pre-post" [tiab] OR "pre test" [tiab] OR "pre-test" [tiab] OR "pretest" [tiab] OR "post test" [tiab] OR "post-test" [tiab]) OR ((before[tiab] AND after [tiab]) OR (before [tiab] AND during [tiab])) OR (quasi-experiment*[tiab] OR quasiexperiment*[tiab] OR quasirandom* [tiab] OR quasi random*[tiab] OR quasicontrol* [tiab] OR quasi control* [tiab]) OR ("time series" [tiab] AND interrupt* [tiab]) OR ("time points" [tiab] AND (multiple[tiab] OR three[tiab] OR four[tiab] OR five[tiab] OR six[tiab] OR seven[tiab] OR eight[tiab] OR nine[tiab] OR ten[tiab] OR month*[tiab] OR hour*[tiab] OR day*[tiab])) OR ("process assessment (health care)" [MeSH Terms] OR program evaluation [mesh]) OR ((clinical [tiab] AND trial [tiab]) OR clinical trials [MeSH Terms] OR clinical trial [Publication Type] OR random*[tiab] OR random allocation [MeSH Terms] OR therapeutic use [MeSH Subheading])	3564636
4	Combine results	#1 AND #2 AND #3	
5	Apply limits	**LIMITS:** English and Human and Adult	1058

APPENDIX B. STUDY SELECTION FORM

Criteria for inclusion and exclusion of studies

Inclusion criteria:

- Study designs recommended by the Cochrane Effective Practice and Organization of Care Group (does NOT include cross-over or observational):
    - Patient or cluster RCTs
    - Nonrandomized cluster controlled trials: An experimental study in which practices or clinicians are allocated to interventions using nonrandom methods
    - Controlled before-and-after studies: A study in which observations are made before and after the implementation of an intervention, both in a group that receives the intervention and in a control group that does not
    - Interrupted time series designs: A study that uses observations at multiple time points before and after an intervention – an attempt to detect if the intervention has had an effect significantly greater than any underlying trend over time

- Sample population has schizophrenia, schizoaffective disorder and/or bipolar disorder, or meets the definition of SMI based on low functional status and least 25% are diagnosed with schizophrenia, schizoaffective disorder and/or bipolar disorder.

- Sample population age 18 and over

- Outpatient population (from mental health clinics and satellite clinics, not community sites)

- Intervention or "exposure" meets definition for integrated care with the explicitly stated goal of improving general medical outcome(s). At a minimum, integrated care must:
    - Involve system redesign such that care providers are added to directly address or coordinate mental and general medical care. Examples include: adding a general medical provider (PA, APN, MD) to the mental health setting, adding a behavioral health specialist who can address multiple behaviors related to general medical care or a health coach /educator /nurse to coordinate and follow through on general medical care with providers located outside the mental health specialty setting.
    - If system redesign with care providers is not used, there must be at least 3 **of the following elements** designed to provide integrated mental and general medical care (decision support, information systems, self-management support, teams care or enhanced communication).

- Includes results on at least one of the relevant outcomes (KQs 1–3)

- Study duration of at least 3 months

- Must be in a peer-reviewed publication

- English language

- Study conducted in North America, Western Europe, Australia/New Zealand

Exclusion criteria:

- Non-English language publication

- Cross-sectional studies and other observational study designs not specifically listed as "included" study designs

- Studies in which the sample is selected for individuals with substance abuse disorders

- Community, rather than practice-based interventions (i.e., not interested in senior centers, but what can be achieved within existing VA clinics and satellite facilities)

- Interventions designed to affect only one specific outcome or aspect of general medical health (e.g., weight loss or smoking cessation, etc.)

- Interventions that involve only: self-management support, enhanced information systems (e.g. EMR, shared records), decision support (e.g., clinical guidelines, clinical reminders) or enhanced access (e.g., location closer to target population or open access scheduling).

APPENDIX C. CRITERIA USED IN QUALITY ASSESSMENT

General Instructions:

For each risk of bias item, rate as "Yes," "No," or "Unclear." After considering each of the quality items, give the study an overall quality rating of good, fair, or poor.

Detailed Quality Items:

If an item is rated as "No," describe why in the comments column.

1. *Randomization adequate?* Was the allocation sequence adequately generated? **Yes/No/Unclear**
2. *Allocation concealment adequate?* Was allocation adequately concealed? **Yes/No/Unclear**
3. *Incomplete outcome data adequately addressed?* **Yes/No/Unclear**
   Consider Attrition bias: Were there systematic differences between groups in withdrawals from a study or high overall loss to followup? (Even small differences could be important when rates are low.) Were subjects excluded from the analysis – if so, were the exclusions sensible?
4. Subjects Blinded? Were subjects blind to treatment assignment? **Yes/No/Unclear**
5. Outcome assessor blinded? (This may be recorded separately for each critically important outcome.) Were Outcome assessors blind to treatment assignment? **Yes/No/Unclear**
6. Provider (treating clinician) blinded? Were providers blind to treatment assignment? **Yes/No/Unclear**
7. All outcomes reported? Are reports of the study free of suggestion of selective outcome reporting (systematic differences between reported and unreported findings)? **Yes/No/Unclear**
8. Intention-to-treat analysis? **Yes** (all eligible patients that were randomized are included in analysis; note- mixed models and survival analyses are in general ITT) **/No/Unclear**
9. *Adequate power for main effects?* **Yes** (if power analysis or sample size calculation given and recruitment met needs or if post-hoc power calculation shows adequate power)**/No** (did not meet projected sample size needs) **/Unclear** (no power or sample size calculation given)
10. *Other Selection bias?* Were there methods that could lead to differences or were there systematic differences observed in baseline characteristics and prognostic factors of the groups compared? (e.g., failure of randomization): **Yes/No/Unclear**
11. Comparable groups maintained? (Includes crossovers, adherence, and contamination.) Consider issues of crossover (e.g., from one intervention to another), adherence (major differences in adherence to the interventions being compared), contamination (e.g., some members of control group get intervention) Yes/No/Unclear
12. *Lack of Performance bias?* Were there no important systematic differences in the care that was provided, other than the intervention of interest? **Yes/No/Unclear**
13. *Lack of Measurement bias?* Were the measures used reliable and valid – and therefore, "yes" no important measurement bias? **Yes/No/Unclear**
14. *Absence of Detection bias?* Were there systematic differences between groups in how outcomes are determined? If no systematic differences answer "yes" – no important detection bias. **Yes/No/Unclear**
15. *Was there the absence of potential important conflict of interest?* The focus here is financial conflict of interest. Therefore if no financial conflict of interest (e.g. funded by government or foundation and authors do not have financial relationships with drug/device manufacturer), then answer "yes." **Yes/No/Unclear**

Overall rating

Please assign each study an overall quality rating of "Good," "Fair," or "Poor" based on the following definitions:

A "**Good**" study has the least bias, and results are considered valid. A good study has a clear description of the population, setting, interventions, and comparison groups; uses a valid approach to allocate patients to alternative treatments; has a low dropout rate; and uses appropriate means to prevent bias, measure outcomes, and analyze and report results.

A "**Fair**" study is susceptible to some bias but probably not enough to invalidate the results. The study may be missing information, making it difficult to assess limitations and potential problems. As the fair-quality category is broad, studies with this rating vary in their strengths and weaknesses. The results of some fair-quality studies are possibly valid, while others are probably valid.

A "**Poor**" rating indicates significant bias that may invalidate the results. These studies have serious errors in design, analysis, or reporting; have large amounts of missing information; or have discrepancies in reporting. The results of a poor-quality study are at least as likely to reflect flaws in the study design as to indicate true differences between the compared interventions.

Table 11. Quality assessment for the four RCTs

Quality item	Druss et al., 2001	Bauer et al., 2006 and Kilbourne et al., 2009	Kilbourne et al., 2008	Druss et al., 2010
1. Randomization adequate?	Yes	Yes	Yes	Yes
2. Allocation concealment adequate?	Unclear	Unclear	Yes	Yes
3. Incomplete outcome date adequately addressed?	Yes	Yes	Yes	Yes
4. Subject blinded?	No	No	Yes	No
5. Outcome assessor blinded?	Unclear	Unclear	Yes	Yes
6. Provider blinded?	No	No	No	No
7. All outcomes reported?	Yes	Yes	Yes	Yes
8. Intention-to-treat analysis?	Yes	Yes	Yes	Yes
9. Adequate power for main effects?	Unclear	Yes	Unclear	Unclear
10. Other selection bias?	Yes	Yes	Yes	Yes
11. Comparable groups maintained?	Yes	Yes	Yes	Yes
12. Lack of performance bias?	Yes	Yes	Yes	Yes
13. Lack of measurement bias?	Yes	Yes	Yes	Yes
14. Absence of detection bias?	Yes	Yes	Yes	Yes
15. Was there the absence of potential important conflict of interest?	Yes	Yes	Yes	Yes

APPENDIX D. PEER REVIEW COMMENTS/AUTHOR RESPONSES

Reviewer	Comment	Response
Question 1: Are the objectives, scope, and methods for this review clearly described?		
1	Yes	Acknowledged
2	Yes. The report is very clear.	Thank you.
3	Yes	Acknowledged
4	Yes	Acknowledged
5	Yes	Acknowledged
Question 2: Is there any indication of bias in our synthesis of the evidence?		
1	No	Acknowledged
2	No	Acknowledged
3	No	Acknowledged
4	No. It is interesting that three out of the four RCTs were VA studies. While I don't think this indicates bias, I think it does reflect the high quality research being conducted in VA and the cutting-edge nature of what VA does. I'm not sure I agree with the statement that this might impact the applicability of the findings to a non-VA setting, although I appreciate the authors' sensitivity to this issue. The fact that two of the four studies included people with bipolar disorder exclusively is a significant limitation, as was pointed out in the review but gives clear direction for future research and emphasizes the need for VA to use a clear definition for "serious mental illness."	Thank you.
5	No	Acknowledged
Question 3: Are there any studies of interest to the VA that we have overlooked?		
1	Not sure: check this one (I will attach pdf to response email): Miller AL, Crismon ML, Rush AJ, et al. The Texas Medication Algorithm project: Clinical results for schizophrenia. Schizophr Bull. 2004;30(3):627-647.	Thank you for the suggestion, but the Miller study would not have met our inclusion criteria for two reasons: (1) The intervention did not meet our definition for integrated care. (2) The purpose was to improve symptoms of schizophrenia, not medical outcomes. The only nonpsychological measure is the SF-12.
2	No. Not to my knowledge	Acknowledged

Reviewer	Comment	Response
3	Yes. Zappe C, Danton W. Integrated mental health and primary care: a model of coordinated services. Federal Practitioner, 2004. June: 74-81. McGuire J, Gelberg L, Blue-Howells J, Rosenheck RA. Access to primary care for homeless veterans with serious mental illness or substance abuse: a follow-up evaluation of co-located primary care and homeless social services. Adm Policy Ment Health, 2009. 36(4): 255-64. Note: neither meets criteria (first for design, 2nd for proportion of participants with SMI) but might be listed under those reports reviewed but not included	Thank you for the suggestions. The Zappe study did not come up in our literature search because it is not an RCT or other included study design. The McGuire study was found in our literature review but was excluded at the abstract level for population not of interest due to substance abuse. Per systematic review standard protocol, it was not included in the table of excluded studies because it was not reviewed at the full-text level.
4	No	Acknowledged
5	Yes. This is likely, given the current interest in PACT and special populations. The review methodology clearly disqualified QI studies in favor of RCTs. While this has scientific merit, it risks overlooking important and usually unfunded pre/post studies. It is, of course, difficult to get QI projects published, so the search for successful interventions would be difficult and at variance from the usual processes and definitions of "evidence synthesis."	We agree that valuable information may be contained in quality improvement evaluations of interventions, many of which do not get published. For the purposes of this review, we used the study criteria recommended in the Cochrane Effective Practice and Organization of Care Search. The established criteria for the evidence synthesis included study designs in addition to RCTs; however, we did not identify any non-RCT studies that met the established criteria.
Question 4: Please write additional suggestions or comments below. If applicable, please indicate the page and line numbers from the draft report.		
1	1. Overall very nice job—hard digging for a few nuggets. Important that you point this out to the field. I particularly like that you have policy/funding directives at the end that are fairly specific, not just "more research is needed." I also like that you list the excluded studies. It allowed me to cross-check our own review quickly and see if there was anything we got that you didn't. It's also great that you list the clinicaltrials.gov list of trials in progress so we can watch for "coming attractions."	Thank you.
	2. Related to this, you have on p 13 a separate section on "Rating the Body of Evidence" but I don't see that as an integral and major part of your Recommendations on p 36. I may have missed it, but this may be because it needs further highlighting.	Text has been added to the Summary and Discussion section about the rating of evidence.
	3. You may want to consider adopting the PRISMA reporting system for your ESPs: Liberati A, Altman DG, Tetzlaff J, et al. The PRISMA statement for reporting systematic reviews and meta-analyses of studies that evaluate health care interventions: Explanation and elaboration. J Clin Epidemiol. 2009;62(10):e1-34; you get the info mostly there but PRISMA is becoming the standard (eg, by JAMA)	Acknowledged

Reviewer	Comment	Response
1 (cont.)	4. It seems that a very key and important issue is that "None of the four trials provided information on general medical outcomes" (p 29 para 3). It seems this should be the #1 focus for future research. I'm not so concerned that a wide variety of care models haven't been tested—it's a good thing that we can build off of one so strongly supported as the CCM. But at this point we really have no idea whether we can make a dent in the deficits that motivated this review in the first place: premature mortality and poor medical outcome.	We agree and have addressed this point in the first paragraph of the Recommendations for Future Research section.
	5. There is a mis-statement on p 29 in para 4 (that is not consistently made in the document but should be corrected here: "Three of the four studies (54-56, 58, 60) evaluated interventions implemented at only one site." References 55, 56, and 58 refer to an 11-site, 3-year RCT.	The reviewer is correct. We simply referenced the wrong study as being the third of the three studies conducted at one site. The two Druss studies are correct. We have replaced the references with Kilbourne 2008.
	6. The exclusion of PTSD as an SMI seems to me to be influenced by programmatic/policy perspectives rather than clinical. To wit: The VA counts as SMI bipolar spectrum and schizophrenia spectrum disorders, but not PTSD; the latter has its own tracking system, clinical programs, and champions who by and large differ from those committed to SMI. However, clinically, PTSD is also typically treated in the specialty MH sector, and medication such as second generation antipsychotics which can worsen medical health are used widely. Thus PTSD is characterized by both fragmentation of care and elevated iatrogenic medical risk. Additionally, more Veterans with PTSD are treated annually by VHA (~300K) than with bipolar disorder (~100K) or schizophrenia (~90K) at last count. On the other hand, most published data on "SMI" focus on the narrower definition that you adopt. In either event, if you go back and look for PTSD it's not likely you'll find any studies, although this one may make it: Zatzick D, Roy-Byrne P, Russo J, et al. A randomized effectiveness trial of stepped collaborative care for acutely injured trauma survivors. Arch Gen Psychiatry. 2004;61(5):498.	We agree that PTSD is an extremely important diagnostic entity, particularly in the VA, and acknowledge the similarities with the disorders emphasized in this review. Diagnostic inclusion criteria were informed by the views of our identified stakeholders. Two of the included studies did have subjects with PTSD. The study cited in the comment is on subjects with PTSD due to physical assault. Some are hospitalized. A good proportion have substance abuse. There are no medical outcomes. While it is an important study, it does not meet the criteria established for this review.
	7. It is likely worth noting that CCMs have begun to enter the clinical practice guideline literature as a fundamental approach to care for SMI—specifically bipolar disorder. Here are two instances, and I believe the draft of the American Psychiatric Association Guideline for bipolar disorder will cite the model as well: VA-DoD: Department of Veterans Affairs & Department of Defense. Clinical practice guideline for management of bipolar disorder in adults, version 2.0. Department of Veterans Affairs Office of Quality and Performance & US Army MEDCOM Quality Management Division. 2009. CANMAT: Yatham LN, Kennedy SH, O'Donovan C, et al. Canadian Network for Mood and Anxiety Treatments (CANMAT) guidelines for the management of patients with bipolar disorder: Update 2007. Bipolar Disord. 2006;8(6):721-739	We have added mention of these guidelines in the summary and discussion of KQ 4.

Reviewer	Comment	Response
2	No specific suggestions/comments.	Acknowledged
3	The report is surprisingly lengthy given the paucity of literature on the topic. It is, however, comprehensive, and detailed on the information that is available. A less restrictive selection strategy may have allowed for more comment (though perhaps in a less definitive manner) on "real world" application of these care models (see 5th item on Table 8, page 29).	Acknowledged
4	While I understand the definition of "integrated care" used in the review, I would not have included "health coach/educator," especially when it comes to providing primary care to individuals with SMI. From my experience, such providers are unprepared to work with individuals with highly complex mental health needs. In addition, "coordinate and follow through" services are qualitatively different from directly providing primary care services in specialty mental health or mental health services in primary care. Including a "health coach/educator" in the definition unnecessarily complicates the issue.	We agree that working with individuals with SMI requires a complex set of skills. The type of health professionals noted in this comment would not provide primary care services to the exclusion of other team members in the models included. We defined the features of integrated care using the chronic care model and medical home model as guides. Therefore, our inclusion criterion for the intervention was, "... meets definition for integrated care with the explicitly stated goal of improving general medical outcome(s). At a minimum, integrated care must: (1) Involve system redesign such that care providers are added to directly address or coordinate mental and general medical care. Examples include: adding a general medical provider (PA, APN, MD) to the mental health setting, adding a behavioral health specialist who can address multiple behaviors related to general medical care ... or a health coach/educator/nurse to coordinate and follow through on general medical care with providers located outside the mental health specialty setting ..."
4	The future directions section seems very much on target. Just as studying the addition of primary care services to Assertive Community Treatment programs could yield interesting findings, so too could the addition of primary care services to Psychosocial Rehabilitation and Recovery Centers, which is another piece of the continuum of care from inpatient to outpatient care. This review is very timely, as OMHS is working to define the interaction of primary care and specialty mental health.	Thank you. We have added mention of PRRCs to the Recommendations for Future Research section.

Reviewer	Comment	Response
5	KQ 4 is the most important question for a developing field of knowledge. RCT evidence to date is so limited that it is difficult to make any conclusions other than "we need to know more." These studies have demonstrated that directly addressing general medical needs in the mental health setting is associated with better processes of care that should lead to better outcomes (we also know that improved health outcomes may not be apparent in the timeline associated with RCTs). Given the dearth of information, the literature to date can best be used to confidently state that doing something is better than doing nothing.	We agree with the points in this comment.
	Given the variability (Kilbourne, Post et al. 2008) in defining "Serious Mental Illness," we need agreement about a research definition of the term that can be applied across future studies.	
	The review notes, but does not emphasize the apparent lack of focus on providing PCMH services within existing/developing PCMH (PACT) programs. Does this imply an assumption that it cannot be done? Are there specific interventions that can assure that patients with SMI can receive care in a VA PACT? Creating SMI PACTS in VA mental health services may be possible in a research environment but is likely to be financially unsustainable. SCAN/ECHO is a model that suggests that, with the right supports/education/mentoring in place, general medical practices can successfully treat complex populations.	We do not assume that PACT cannot successfully address the needs of individuals with SMI. The studies reviewed had a treatment-as-usual condition that was not consistent with PACT even though 3 of 4 studies did occur in the VA. We have added text to the KQ 1 discussion to reflect uncertainty about whether PACT can work with individuals with SMI.
5	There is also need to explore models useful in CBOCs. Many CBOCs, by virtue of their small size, have developed fully integrated care programs, though without calling them programs. There is likely a wealth of information about what has been helpful, that could then be tested in RCTs.	We have added some discussion of CBOCs in the Recommendations for Future Research section.

Question 5. Are there any clinical performance measures, programs, quality improvement measures, patient care services, or conferences that will be directly affected by this report? If so, please provide detail.

Reviewer	Comment	Response
1	The Mental Health QUERI SMI Health Work Group will be very interested in this (Dr. Williams is a member so I'm sure they will be in the loop).	Acknowledged
2	As the report indicates, this evidence synthesis is highly relevant to the Patient Centered Medical Home (PACT) initiative. This report will be immensely useful to the strategic planning of the Mental Health QUERI SMI Health Workgroup.	Thank you.
3	Not directly	Acknowledged
4	No comment	Acknowledged
5	The Primary Care – Mental Health Integration program has had its lens focused almost entirely on provision of MH services in PC. These services have been mostly limited to care of common, relatively straightforward psychological, psychiatric and social problems. This report may be helpful in expanding those horizons. Likewise, the added emphasis on the patient population most likely to negatively impact on any given PACT performance measure will be important. The studies reviewed note very specific target conditions, which are good fodder for local QI initiatives	Acknowledged

Reviewer	Comment	Response
Question 6: Please provide any recommendations on how this report can be revised to more directly address or assist implementation needs.		
1	1. CCMs per se are really not on the radar of OMHS and this report indicates that they should be. 2. This report also highlights the need for better tracking of quality of care processes for SMI Veterans. Specifically, there have been overlapping/colliding efforts across OMHS and OQP to develop performance measures around metabolic monitoring and SMI (with/without antipsychotic use). Amy Kilbourne was leading this nascent effort that I think has, unfortunately, died on the vine. I would hope that the recommendations of this report might reinvigorate this effort.	Acknowledged
2	No revisions are needed.	Thank you.
3	Unfortunately, the literature review suggest benefits but, as laid out clearly in the report, there are many gaps remaining in knowledge on this topic.	Acknowledged
4	No comment	Acknowledged
5	Like the AHRQ funded reports a few years ago, cautioning against "premature orthodoxy" is important.	We have added text to address this in the KQ 4 discussion.
Question 7: Please provide us with contact details of any additional individuals/stakeholders who should be made aware of this report.		
1	Not sure who you are already going to contact. The Usual Suspects probably include MH QUERI and OMHS. Diabetes QUERI and related medically oriented QUERIs also come to mind. OQP (or whatever it's called now) Grant Huang the head of CSP, since you recommend a CSP-level trial The SMI Committee in particular under OMHS Outside VA: NAMI and the Depression & Bipolar Support Alliance	Thank you for the suggestions. We will disseminate the report in these directions.
2	I believe the key stakeholders have already been included in developing this report, including OMHS, HSR&D/QUERI, and Mental Health QUERI. The Primary Care-Mental Health Integration Initiative and PACT leaders should be made aware if they are not already on the list.	Thank you for the suggestions. We will disseminate the report in these directions.
3	No comment	Acknowledged
4	No comment	Acknowledged
5	Jeff Burk, national director of psychosocial rehab and recovery is vital to this area. If not already reviewing, he should be added	Thank you for the suggestion. Dr. Burk was a reviewer of this report. We will make sure he is aware of the final report.

APPENDIX E. EXCLUDED STUDIES

All studies listed below were reviewed in their full-text version and excluded for the reason indicated. An alphabetical reference list follows the table.

Reference	Not SMI	Not outpatient	Not RCT	Not integrated care	No medical outcomes	Not peer-reviewed	Not Westernized culture
Adair et al., 2005 (1039)			X				
Baker et al., 2009 (1055)			X				
Bauer et al., 2001 (1592)				X			
Bauer et al., 2007 (1558)						X	
Byng et al., 2004 (434)					X		
Chafetz et al., 2008 (152)		X					
Chiverton et al., 2007 (185)	X						
Ciompi et al., 1992 (907)			X				
Davies et al., 2008 (1134)			X				
Desai et al., 2002 (16)	X						
Desai et al., 2002 (23)	X						
Dewa et al., 2009 (82)	X						
Dickerson et al., 2003 (11)			X				
Donald et al., 2005 (395)			X				
Drew et al., 2007 (217)			X				
Druss et al., 2010 (21)				X			
Essock et al., 1998 (687)					X		
Essock et al., 1995 (820)					X		
Essock et al., 2006 (319)				X			
Forsberg et al., 2008 (1553)				X			
Harvey et al., 2005 (1200)				X			
Jerrell et al., 1995 (806)					X		
Kahn et al., 2009 (46)	X						
Kalichman et al., 1995 (832)				X			

Reference	Not SMI	Not outpatient	Not RCT	Not integrated care	No medical outcomes	Not peer-reviewed	Not Westernized culture
Katon et al., 1991 (929)	X						
Kemp et al., 2010 (1234)				X			
Know et al., 2006 (1267)							X
Madhusoodanam et al., 2006 (1298)			X				
Malla et al., 1998 (675)				X			
McKibbin et al., 2010 (1324)				X			
Ohlsen et al., 2005 (341)			X				
O'Kearney et al., 2004 (1362)			X				
Pirraglia et al., 2009 (1380)			X				
Poulin et al., 2007 (1383)				X			
Ridgely et al., 1996 (774)			X				
Rivera et al., 2007 (225)				X			
Robson et al., 1984 (960)	X						
Rubin et al., 2005 (376)		X					
Ryan et al., 2007 (207)	X						
Sartorius et al., 1993 (887)	X						
Sata et al., 1999 (614)	X						
Schmidt-Kraepelin et al., 2009 (55)					X		
Sim et al., 2006 (1446)				X			
Simon et al., 2006 (1694)				X			
Snyder et al., 2008 (1693)				X			
Symonds et al., 2007 (1692)	X						
Taborda et al., 2003 (471)						X	
Thompson et al., 2006 (1484)				X			
Welch et al., 2009 (84)			X				
Wright et al., 2006 (308)			X				

LIST OF EXCLUDED STUDIES

Adair CE, McDougall GM, Mitton CR, et al. Continuity of Care and Health Outcomes Among Persons With Severe Mental Illness. *Psychiatr Serv*. 2005;56(9):1061-1069.

Baker A, Richmond R, Castle D, et al. Coronary heart disease risk reduction intervention among overweight smokers with a psychotic disorder: Pilot trial. *Aust N Z J Psychiatry*. 2009;43(2):129-135.

Bauer MS. The collaborative practice model for bipolar disorder: design and implementation in a multi-site randomized controlled trial. *Bipolar Disorders*; 2001:233-44.

Bauer Ms KAM. Outcome and Costs in a Randomized Controlled Effectiveness Trial of a Collaborative Chronic Care Model for Bipolar Disorder. *Journal of Mental Health Policy and Economics*; 2007:S3.

Byng R, Jones R, Leese M, et al. Exploratory cluster randomised controlled trial of shared care development for long-term mental illness. *Br J Gen Pract*. 2004;54(501):259-66.

Chafetz L, White M, Collins-Bride G, et al. Clinical trial of wellness training: health promotion for severely mentally ill adults. *J Nerv Ment Dis*. 2008;196(6):475-83.

Chiverton P, Lindley P, Tortoretti DM, et al. Well balanced: 8 steps to wellness for adults with mental illness and diabetes. *J Psychosoc Nurs Ment Health Serv*. 2007;45(11):46-55.

Ciompi L, Dauwalder HP, Maier C, et al. The pilot project 'Soteria Berne'. Clinical experiences and results. *Br J Psychiatry Suppl*. 1992(18):145-53.

Davies LM, Barnes TRE, Jones PB, et al. A randomized controlled trial of the cost-utility of second-generation antipsychotics in people with psychosis and eligible for clozapine. *Value in Health*. 2008;11(4):549-562.

Desai MM, Rosenheck RA, Druss BG, et al. Mental disorders and quality of care among postacute myocardial infarction outpatients. *J Nerv Ment Dis*. 2002;190(1):51-3.

Desai MM, Rosenheck RA, Druss BG, et al. Receipt of nutrition and exercise counseling among medical outpatients with psychiatric and substance use disorders. *J Gen Intern Med*. 2002;17(7):556-60.

Dewa CS, Hoch JS, Carmen G, et al. Cost, effectiveness, and cost-effectiveness of a collaborative mental health care program for people receiving short-term disability benefits for psychiatric disorders. *Can J Psychiatry*. 2009;54(6):379-88.

Dickerson FB, McNary SW, Brown CH, et al. Somatic healthcare utilization among adults with serious mental illness who are receiving community psychiatric services. *Med Care*. 2003;41(4):560-70.

Donald M, Dower J, Kavanagh D. Integrated versus non-integrated management and care for clients with co-occurring mental health and substance use disorders: a qualitative systematic review of randomised controlled trials. *Soc Sci Med*. 2005;60(6):1371-83.

Drew L, Delacy F. Improving the general health of persons with psychosis. *Australas Psychiatry*. 2007;15(4):320-3.

Druss BG, Zhao L, von Esenwein SA, et al. The Health and Recovery Peer (HARP) Program: A peer-led intervention to improve medical self-management for persons with serious mental illness. *Schizophr Res*. 2010.

Essock SM, Frisman LK, Kontos NJ. Cost-effectiveness of assertive community treatment teams. *Am J Orthopsychiatry*. 1998;68(2):179-90.

Essock SM, Kontos N. Implementing assertive community treatment teams. *Psychiatr Serv*. 1995;46(7):679-83.

Essock SM, Mueser KT, Drake RE, et al. Comparison of ACT and standard case management for delivering integrated treatment for co-occurring disorders. *Psychiatr Serv*. 2006;57(2):185-96.

Forsberg KA, Björkman T, Sandman PO, et al. Physical health--a cluster randomized controlled lifestyle intervention among persons with a psychiatric disability and their staff. *Nordic Journal of Psychiatry*; 2008:486-95.

Harvey SB, Newton A, Moye GA. Physical health monitoring in schizophrenia: The use of an invitational letter in a primary care setting. *Primary Care & Community Psychiatry*. 2005;10(2):71-74.

Jerrell JM, Ridgely MS. Gender differences in the assessment of specialized treatments for substance abuse among people with severe mental illness. *J Psychoactive Drugs*. 1995;27(4):347-55.

Kahn LS, Fox CH, Carrington J, et al. Telephonic nurse case management for patients with diabetes and mental illnesses: a qualitative perspective. *Chronic Illn*. 2009;5(4):257-67.

Kalichman SC, Sikkema KJ, Kelly JA, et al. Use of a brief behavioral skills intervention to prevent HIV infection among chronic mentally ill adults. *Psychiatr Serv*. 1995;46(3):275-80.

Katon WJ. The development of a randomized trial of consultation-liaison psychiatry trial in distressed high utilizers of primary care. *Psychiatr Med*. 1991;9(4):577-91.

Kemp DE, Gao K, Chan PK, et al. Medical comorbidity in bipolar disorder: Relationship between illnesses of the endocrine metabolic system and treatment outcome. *Bipolar Disorders*. 2010;12(4):404-413.

Kwon JS, Choi J-S, Bahk W-M, et al. Weight Management Program for Treatment-Emergent Weight Gain in Olanzapine-Treated Patients With Schizophrenia or Schizoaffective Disorder: A 12-Week Randomized Controlled Clinical Trial. *J Clin Psychiatry*. 2006;67(4):547-553.

Madhusoodanan S, Moise D, Sajatovic M. Schizoaffective disorder in the elderly. In: French DP, ed. *Schizophrenic psychology: New research*. Hauppauge, NY US: Nova Science Publishers; 2006:57-82.

Malla AK, Norman RM, McLean TS, et al. An integrated medical and psychosocial treatment program for psychotic disorders: patient characteristics and outcome. *Can J Psychiatry*. 1998;43(7):698-705.

McKibbin CL, Golshan S, Griver K, et al. A healthy lifestyle intervention for middle-aged and older schizophrenia patients with diabetes mellitus: A 6-month follow-up analysis. *Schizophr Res*. 2010;121(1-3):203-206.

Ohlsen RI, Peacock G, Smith S. Developing a service to monitor and improve physical health in people with serious mental illness. *J Psychiatr Ment Health Nurs*. 2005;12(5):614-9.

O'Kearney R, Garland G, Welch M, et al. Factors predicting program fidelity and delivery of an early intervention program for first episode psychosis in rural Australia. *AeJAMH (Australian e-Journal for the Advancement of Mental Health)*. 2004;3(2).

Pirraglia PA, Biswas K, Kilbourne AM, et al. A prospective study of the impact of comorbid medical disease on bipolar disorder outcomes. *J Affect Disord*. 2009;115(3):355-359.

Poulin M-J, Chaput J-P, Simard V, et al. Management of antipsychotic-induced weight gain: Prospective naturalistic study of the effectiveness of a supervised exercise programme. *Aust N Z J Psychiatry*. 2007;41(12):980-989.

Ridgely MS, Morrissey JP, Paulson RI, et al. Characteristics and activities of case managers in the RWJ Foundation Program on chronic mental illness. *Psychiatr Serv*. 1996;47(7):737-43.

Rivera JJ, Sullivan AM, Valenti SS. Adding consumer-providers to intensive case management: does it improve outcome? *Psychiatr Serv*. 2007;58(6):802-9.

Robson MH, France R, Bland M. Clinical psychologist in primary care: controlled clinical and economic evaluation. *Br Med J (Clin Res Ed)*. 1984;288(6433):1805-8.

Rubin AS, Littenberg B, Ross R, et al. Effects on processes and costs of care associated with the addition of an internist to an inpatient psychiatry team. *Psychiatr Serv*. 2005;56(4):463-7.

Ryan T, Hatfield B, Sharma I. Outcomes of referrals over a six-month period to a mental health gateway team. *J Psychiatr Ment Health Nurs*. 2007;14(6):527-34.

Sartorius N, Ustun TB, Costa e Silva JA, et al. An international study of psychological problems in primary care. Preliminary report from the World Health Organization Collaborative Project on 'Psychological Problems in General Health Care'. *Arch Gen Psychiatry*. 1993;50(10):819-24.

Sata M, Yoshitake K, Utsunomiya H, et al. Factors affecting disability in patients attending the internal medicine departments of general hospitals. *Psychiatry Clin Neurosci*. 1999;53(6):611-20.

Schmidt-Kraepelin C, Janssen B, Gaebel W. Prevention of rehospitalization in schizophrenia: results of an integrated care project in Germany. *European Archives of Psychiatry and Clinical Neuroscience*. 2009;259 Suppl 2:S205-12.

Sim K, Chan YH, Chua TH, et al. Physical comorbidity, insight, quality of life and global functioning in first episode schizophrenia: A 24-month, longitudinal outcome study. *Schizophr Res*. 2006;88(1-3):82-89.

Simon GE, Ludman EJ, Bauer MS, et al. Long-term effectiveness and cost of a systematic care program for bipolar disorder. *Arch Gen Psychiatry*. 2006;63(5):500-8.

Snyder K, Dobscha SK, Ganzini L, et al. Clinical outcomes of integrated psychiatric and general medical care. *Community Ment Health J*. 2008;44(3):147-54.

Symonds D, Parker R. The Top End Mental Health Services General Practice Clinic: an initiative for patients with serious mental illness. *Australas Psychiatry*. 2007;15(1):58-61.

Taborda JG, Bordignon S, Bertolote JM, et al. Heart transplantation and schizophrenia. *Psychosomatics*. 2003;44(3):264-5.

Thompson WK, Kupfer DJ, Fagiolini A, et al. Prevalence and Clinical Correlates of Medical Comorbidities in Patients With Bipolar I Disorder: Analysis of Acute-Phase Data From a Randomized Controlled Trial. *J Clin Psychiatry*. 2006;67(5):783-788.

Welch K. GPs have a central role in managing schizophrenia. *Practitioner*. 2009;253(1718):19-23.

Wright CA, Osborn DP, Nazareth I, et al. Prevention of coronary heart disease in people with severe mental illnesses: a qualitative study of patient and professionals' preferences for care. *BMC Psychiatry*. 2006;6:16.

APPENDIX F. GLOSSARY

Abstract screening

The stage in a systematic review during which titles and abstracts of articles identified in the literature search are screened for inclusion or exclusion based on established criteria. Articles that pass the abstract screening stage are promoted to the full-text review stage.

ClinicalTrials.gov

A registry and results database of federally and privately supported clinical trials conducted in the United States and around the world. ClinicalTrials.gov provides information about a trial's purpose, location, participant characteristics, among other details.

Cochrane Database of Systematic Reviews

A bibliographic database of peer-reviewed systematic reviews and protocols prepared by the Cochrane Review Groups in The Cochrane Collaboration.

Companion article

A companion article is a publication from a trial that is not the paper containing the main results of that trial. It may be a methods paper, a report of subgroup analyses, a report of combined analyses, or other auxiliary topic that adds information to the interpretation of the main paper.

Confidence interval (CI)

The range in which a particular result (such as a laboratory test) is likely to occur for everyone who has a disease. "Likely" usually means 95 percent of the time. Clinical research studies are conducted on only a certain number of people with a disease rather than all the people who have the disease. The study's results are true for the people who were in the study but not necessarily for everyone who has the disease. The confidence interval is a statistical estimate of how much the study findings would vary if other different people participated in the study. A confidence interval is defined by two numbers, one lower than the result found in the study and the other higher than the study's result. The size of the confidence interval is the difference between these two numbers.

Data abstraction

The stage of a systematic review that involves a pair of trained researchers extracting reported findings specific to the research questions from the full-text articles that met the established inclusion criteria. These data form the basis of the evidence synthesis.

Exclusion criteria

The criteria, or standards, set out before a study or review. Exclusion criteria are used to determine whether a person should participate in a research study or whether an individual study should be excluded in a systematic review. Exclusion criteria may include age, previous treatments, and other medical conditions.

Full-text review

The stage of a systematic review in which a pair of trained researches evaluates the full-text of study articles for potential inclusion in the review.

GRADE

Grading of Recommendations Assessment, Development and Evaluation (GRADE), a system of assessing the quality of medical evidence and evaluating the strength of recommendations based on the evidence.

Inclusion criteria

The criteria, or standards, set out before the systematic review. Inclusion criteria are used to determine whether an individual study can be included in a systematic review. Inclusion criteria may include population, study design, gender, age, type of disease being treated, previous treatments, and other medical conditions.

Nonrandomized study

Any quantitative study estimating the effectiveness of an intervention (harm or benefit) that does not use randomization to allocate units to comparison groups (including studies where "allocation" occurs in the course of usual treatment decisions or peoples' choices; i.e., studies usually called "observational"). There are many possible types of nonrandomized intervention studies, including cohort studies, case-control studies, controlled before-and-after studies, interrupted-time-series studies, and controlled trials that do not use appropriate randomization strategies (sometimes called quasi-randomised studies).

Observational study

A study in which the investigators do not seek to intervene but simply observe the course of events. Changes or differences in one characteristic (e.g., whether or not people received the intervention of interest) are studied in relation to changes or differences in other characteristics (e.g., whether or not they died), without action by the investigator. Observational studies provide weaker empirical evidence than do experimental studies because of the potential for large confounding biases to be present when there is an unknown association between a factor and an outcome.

PsycINFO®

An abstracting and indexing database of peer-reviewed literature in the behavioral sciences and mental health.

Publication bias

The tendency of researchers to publish experimental findings that have a positive result, while not publishing the findings when the results are negative or inconclusive. The effect of publication bias is that published studies may be misleading. When information that differs from that of the published study is not known, people are able to draw conclusions using only information from the published studies.

PubMed®

A database of citations for biomedical literature from MEDLINE®, life science journals, and online books in the fields of medicine, nursing, dentistry, veterinary medicine, the health care system, and preclinical sciences.

Quasi-experimental study

Often described as a nonrandomized, pre-post intervention study. A study based on a true experimental design meets two criteria: manipulation of a variable factor between two or more groups and random assignment of participants to those groups. A quasi-experimental study uses the first criterion, but participants are not randomly assigned to groups. This means a researcher cannot draw conclusions about cause and effect. Quasi-experimental study designs are frequently used when it is not logistically feasible or ethical to conduct a randomized controlled trial.

Randomized controlled trial

A prospective, analytical, experimental study using primary data generated in the clinical environment. Individuals similar at the beginning of the trial are randomly allocated to two or more treatment groups and the outcomes the groups are compared after sufficient followup time. Properly executed, the RCT is the strongest evidence of the clinical efficacy of preventive and therapeutic procedures in the clinical setting.

Risk

A way of expressing the chance that something will happen. It is a measure of the association between exposure to something and what happens (the outcome). Risk is the same as probability, but it usually is used to describe the probability of an adverse event. It is the rate of events (such as breast cancer) in the total population of people who could have the event (such as women of a certain age).

Serious mental illness (SMI)

Defined in this report according to the definition stipulated in Public Law (P.L.) 102–321; that is, a diagnosable mental, behavioral, or emotional disorder, at some time during the past year, that met the criteria in the *Diagnostic and Statistical Manual of Mental Disorders*, 4th edition (DSM-IV) (American Psychiatric Association, 1994) and resulted in functional impairment that substantially interfered with or limited one or more major life activities.

Statistical significance

A mathematical technique to measure whether the results of a study are likely to be true. Statistical significance is calculated as the probability that an effect observed in a research study is occurring because of chance. Statistical significance is usually expressed as a P-value. The smaller the P-value, the less likely it is that the results are due to chance (and more likely that the results are true). Researchers generally believe the results are probably true if the statistical significance is a P-value less than 0.05 (p<.05).

Strength of evidence (SOE)

A measure of how confident reviewers are about decisions that may be made based on a body of evidence. SOE is evaluated using one of four grades: (1) *High* confidence that the evidence reflects the true effect; further research is very unlikely to change reviewer confidence in the estimate of effect; (2) *moderate* confidence that the evidence reflects the true effect; further research may change the confidence in the estimate of effect and may change the estimate; (3) *low* confidence that the evidence reflects the true effect; further research is likely to change the confidence in the estimate of effect and is likely to change the estimate; and (4) *insufficient*; the evidence either is unavailable or does not permit a conclusion.

Systematic review

A summary of the clinical literature. A systematic review is a critical assessment and evaluation of all research studies that address a particular clinical issue. The researchers use an organized method of locating, assembling, and evaluating a body of literature on a particular topic using a set of specific criteria. A systematic review typically includes a description of the findings of the collection of research studies. The systematic review may also include a quantitative pooling of data, called a meta-analysis.

Time-series study

A quasi-experimental research design in which periodic measurements are made on a defined group of individuals both before and after implementation of an intervention. Time series studies are often conducted for the purpose of determining the intervention or treatment effect.

www.ingramcontent.com/pod-product-compliance
Lightning Source LLC
Chambersburg PA
CBHW081607170526
45166CB00009B/2862